OUTSMART SUGAR

HOW TO RETRAIN YOUR BRAIN TO KICK THE SUGAR HABIT

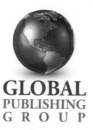

GLOBAL
PUBLISHING
G R O U P

Global Publishing Group
Australia • New Zealand • Singapore • America • London

OUTSMART SUGAR

HOW TO RETRAIN YOUR BRAIN TO KICK THE SUGAR HABIT

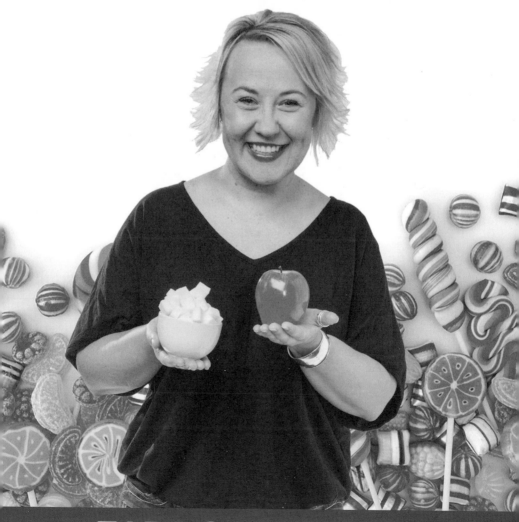

TARA C. MITCHELL

First Edition 2016

Copyright © 2016 Tara Mitchell

National Library of Australia
Cataloguing-in-Publication entry:

Creator: Mitchell, Tara C., author.

Title: Outsmart sugar : how to retrain your brain to kick the sugar habit / Tara C Mitchell.

1st ed.
ISBN: 9781925288070 (paperback)

Subjects: Weight loss.
Self-esteem.
Sugar-free diet.

Dewey Number: 613.25

Published by Global Publishing Group
PO Box 517 Mt Evelyn, Victoria 3796 Australia
Email Info@GlobalPublishingGroup.com.au

Printed in China

For further information about orders:
Phone: +61 3 9739 4686 or Fax +61 3 8648 6871

Dedicated to Toby, the love of my life and my greatest cheerleader. Thank you for always pushing me to get out of my own way!

Also to the Mitchell and Kulinski clans, for instilling in me a fearless approach to life and a love for all things food.

Tara Mitchell

ACKNOWLEDGEMENTS

Wow – what a ride! It's been a life goal for many years for me to write (and finish!) a book and now I've finally done it! Of course, such things don't happen in a vacuum and there are so many people who've inspired and encouraged me along the way.

First and foremost, Thank You to my darling Toby for your tireless work in providing endless hugs and encouragement throughout the book writing process. Also for pouring copious amounts of red wine, metaphorically kicking my butt and constantly instigating huge fits of laughter (even when my head was up my own backside!) – without all these, this book would never have been finished! Shall we get married sometime this decade?

To the amazing team at Global Publishing – Darren, Jackie, Helen, Kelly and Darlene. It's said that everyone has a book in them, but sometimes it's buried so deep it seems it'll never emerge! You guys are the best at extracting books (and thumbs from nether regions!) from all sorts of incredible people who go on to change the world. A special mention to Jackie for helping me cut through the B.S. and nail the book title and to Darren for…Circles!

My love of cooking, gardening and food was instilled from a young age by Mum, Dad and both sets of grandparents. Thank You for teaching me what I consider to be the most important life skills anyone can have. Thank You to incredible chefs like Stephanie Alexander and Jamie Oliver, who take up the cause for other children who weren't quite as lucky as I was, and inspire them to get into the garden and kitchen. I tip my toque to you!

Thank You to Rik Schnabel for your teachings in NLP and for flipping that switch, ridding me of the demon brown liquid forever! To all my fellow CALM'ers, Thank You for baring your souls and being brave enough to share your personal stories with what were a bunch of total strangers. But of course, strangers are just friends we haven't met yet and I'm proud to now call you my buddies for life!

To Sarah Wilson, JJ Virgin, Michelle Bridges, Michelle Tam, Kayla Itsines, Dr Libby, Cynthia Louise and Sarah Taylor: Ladies, I adore and admire your kick-butt attitude towards life and proving that it's not that bloody hard to eat healthily. I salute you!

To Brian Wansink, Damon Gameau, Morgan Spurlock, Pete Evans, Dr Mark Hyman, Bart Baggart, David Gillespie, Tim Ferris, Arnold Schwarzenegger and Paul McKenna: Gents, your expertise and generosity in sharing your passions and knowledge with the world is such an inspiration to me. Thank You!

Most of all, Thank You to You - the reader of this book. Thank You for picking up Outsmart Sugar and making a real commitment to improving your health.

You always have choices in life and the fact that you have chosen this book is truly humbling to me.

Now – go out there and get 'em Tiger!!!

CONTENTS

FREE BONUS GIFT

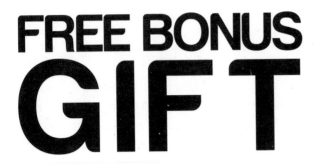
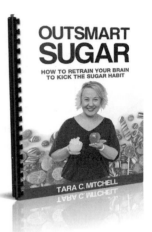

THINK YOU'RE TOO BUSY FOR BREAKFAST?

Visit **www.OutsmartSugarNow.com**
to download your FREE copy of my Top Ten Tips
"How to Outsmart Sugar at Breakfast and Supercharge your Day!"

Plus loads more Resources, Recipes and Ideas
to help you Outsmart Sugar for good!

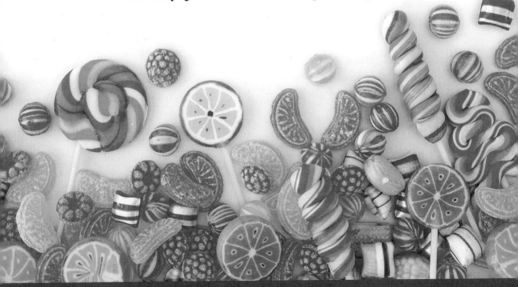

INTRODUCTION

WARNING: This is not a book about deprivation, withdrawal, going cold turkey or "quitting" sugar. It's not about demonising all kinds of sugar either. I know it's very fashionable right now to eliminate sugar entirely, but that seems to have warped the general public's perception of what sugar actually is.

When I talk to many people about my book and the studies that have gone into it, their first question is "But what about fruit?" Indeed, what about fruit? Whole fruit is fantastic stuff – full of fibre, vitamins, minerals and, yes, natural sugar. Nature has a wonderful habit of packaging up perfection like that. It's when we humans start messing with it that things start to go wrong. Naturally occurring sugar shouldn't be of concern to you, but even if you occasionally get stuck into Grandma's triple Chocolate Fudge Cake with Caramel Icing, never ever feel bad about it. Feeling guilty about food choices causes a nasty spiral of self-doubt and insecurity and some people turn to more sugar to fix those feelings!

Feeling great about choosing the best possible whole foods will always, always include the amazing home-made dessert, crafted with heart and soul by someone who truly loves you. It's the processed crap with more numbers on the components list (Food Manufacturers like to call this an "ingredient" list!) than actual, recognisable products that should scare you. If your Grandma wouldn't recognise it, it's not real food.

That said, I won't come around to your office and ruin the staff birthday celebrations by throwing all the birthday cakes in the bin, confiscating your Tim Tams or ferreting out the stash of lollies you have discreetly hidden in your second desk drawer. Don't think I don't know it's there – I used to have one and I know all the strategies and tactics for fooling not only yourself, but your co-workers.

Like me, you think you're being smart – you know as well as I do that your colleagues will rifle through your desk drawers when you're not there, searching for the stapler, sticky-tape, scissors or last pad of Post-it notes. I kept spares of all of these – plus numerous pens, staples, erasers and various other stationery accoutrements – in the first drawer, always the first drawer. This way, you've Outsmarted your colleague who, on the pretence of looking for the elusive stapler (where do those things all go? The same dimension as odd socks, or are there special segments of the hidden universe reserved exclusively for domestic household items and another for office gear?) cannot find your hoarded goodies. They find what they're squirrelling for and move away quickly, nothing to see here.

Your stash is safe… for now.

Nor will I break into your home, extract the step ladder you have stored in that awkward gap between the fridge and the wall, climb up and pull down the blocks of family-sized chocolate you have squirrelled away behind the jars of pasta sauce or "healthy" cereal, so your kids or housemates will never think to look there (trust me, they know it's there). I won't risk frost-bite and rummage around in your freezer, seeking out the mini fun-size chocolates, cleverly disguised in plastic bags that previously housed frozen spinach or beans, and chuck them in the bin.

I'm not interested in finding those bags of lollies stowed in your glove box or centre console of your car, which are only there for "emergencies" when you "need an energy hit". Or the ones in your handbag, supposedly there for the same purpose. You may be wondering why your stashes of sugar don't worry or concern me – isn't this a book about getting rid of unwanted, processed sugar in your life? Indeed it is, but I know that if

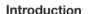

Introduction

you follow the principles I'm about to show you, you won't need me or anyone else to take the sugar away from you. You'll be able to dismiss it easily and effortlessly all on your own.

I know that you're aware on some level, that if someone forces you to "quit" or "give up" something (even if that someone is you!) you feel deprived, disadvantaged and like something's missing. In reality, our Inner Child is still very active when something is taken away from us. Eventually, we will throw a tantrum! It may not be quite as spectacular as the toddler meltdown in aisle four at the Supermarket, but our Inner Child will rebel against the so-called deprivation.

The contents of this book will turn the notion of deprivation on its head. By the end of this book, you won't need me to go commando on you and come around to your house, eliminating anything containing processed sugar. You'll make the healthy choice without even thinking about it, leaving you with ample brain power to focus on other areas of your life.

How do I know this?

Because I've done it.

I went from ice-cream for breakfast and multiple cans of Coke a day, to looking at a can of Coke and thinking "That's a pretty shade of red" and passing by it completely. Yes – it really was as easy as that!

Want to know how? Then read on!

CHAPTER 1

HELLO, MY NAME IS TARA AND I AM A FORMER SUGAR "ADDICT"

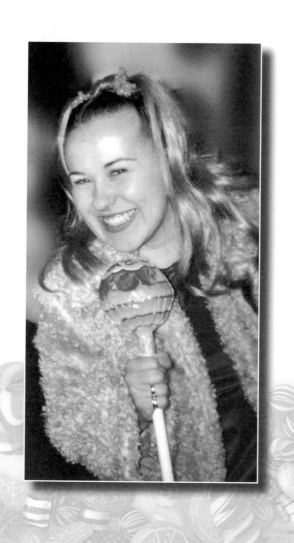

CHAPTER 1

HELLO, MY NAME IS TARA AND I AM A FORMER SUGAR "ADDICT"

This is a picture of me with what I believe is the largest Chupa Chup in the world. I am at a fancy dress party, doing my very best impersonation of Baby Spice (don't judge, it was the early noughties!!).

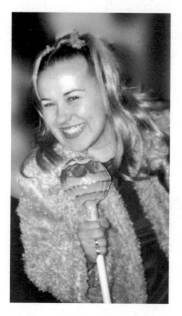

[Tara with Giant Chupa Chup]

I almost had everyone fooled that it was just a prop. But it was 100% real, 100% sugar. You better believe I ate the whole thing. On my own. Without help. I worked as a sales rep for one of the world's largest confectionary companies (you know who they are, they like the colour purple a lot!) a dream job for some, but for me was the equivalent of an alcoholic working at a distillery. I had unfettered access to all manner of chocolate and confectionery – several hundred different lines of products, which of course all had to be taste-tested. No self-respecting sales person refuses to try the product they're selling!

At the time, 40 to 60 new lines were launched every year, using the scattergun approach to consumer marketing. As the saying goes – throw enough mud and some will eventually stick. The confectionary segment is not only about old favourites (although sentimentality plays a big part in food marketing, as well as your personal views on food – more on this later) but also new products, all of which are more exciting, colourful and novel than the last. Of course, not all of them sold well, so someone had to save the boxes and boxes of product from the dump. Not only was my car full of products, but the coffee table at home had a constantly full giant bowl of lollies and chocolates, much to the joy of my housemates and our visitors.

I had unrestricted, totally free access to sugar, 24/7. As I'm sure you know, we tend to put a value on things based on the price we pay for them. As I wasn't paying any money for all this sugar, I never gave it a second thought and it just became my constant companion. I was always very popular at parties, as I'd always bring giant bags of lollies (only available via wholesale, so you can imagine the impressive size), get everyone hyperactive on sugar and amp up the party vibe!

At some point during this sugar-soaked employment, smoothies became very popular. I'd never really been a massive breakfast fan, preferring to grab a (hidden sugar-laden) muesli bar on my way out the door, but this new fad looked right up my alley. Healthy AND portable – what more could a busy girl need? Remember, this was well before the days of green smoothies and juicing, back when low-fat yoghurt was seen as the ideal weight-loss food. When I say that my daily routine consisted of ice-cream for breakfast, I'm sure you're thinking this was just a one-off, maybe a birthday treat or holiday indiscretion. This is the actual recipe for my 'healthy' morning smoothie:

Ingredients

- 1 x large banana, peeled and chopped

- 1.5 cups of low-fat milk

- 2 very large scoops (OK, half a container!) of vanilla ice-cream

Method

Put all ingredients into metal milkshake container, blend 'til smooth with stick blender. Rinse stick blender under tap. Run out door with "healthy" breakfast in hand.

Here was my logic at the time:

- Bananas - fruit, so of course that's healthy, duh!

- Milk – low-fat of course, and absolutely essential for bone health. My grandmother suffered terribly from osteoporosis and I thought I could ward it off by consuming vast amounts of dairy.

- Ice cream – my tastebuds had become so desensitised to sugar, that the banana and lactose in the milk didn't even register on the sweetness scale for me, nor was it creamy enough. This was in the dark ages before I came across the revolutionary idea that freezing chunks of banana made an amazing difference when thrown into a blender. Therefore, a couple of huge scoops of ice-cream seemed like the perfect solution.

Every. Single. Day.

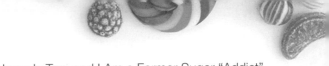

Knowing what I know now, and is totally obvious to you, I can see that I had set myself up for massive failure throughout the day. Once the immense sugar rush of the "healthy" smoothie had worn off, I crashed into the depths of sugar withdrawal. Being the logical, university-educated person I am, the empirical evidence that a hit of sugar got me the energy in the first place led to the logical conclusion… that more sugar was the only solution to getting me back there. So the first bag of lollies was opened and kept at my side for the day. I mindlessly picked at it and was constantly surprised at the end of the day when there was an empty wrapper on the passenger seat of the car. Sometimes two.

Every. Single. Day.

Not long after that, I made the smart move to another employer. Somewhat out of the frying pan and into the fryer – I started work at a wine wholesaler. Yet another 'dream' job some might say. Which I did! I had a lot of fun, what with the interesting and varied clientele I had – restaurant and cafe owners, directors of multi-national hotel groups, not to mention the extravagant events (degustation dinners with one of the best French champagne houses? Tick! Being picked up by helicopter for an aerial vineyard tour before being deposited in the middle of it for a night of sumptuous fully-catered glamping? Tick!) Glamorous though it sounded, and actually was at times, the late nights and long hours on the road took their toll. I didn't have my sugar and chocolate "staff benefits" to keep me going (and consuming my current "staff benefits" whilst driving was illegal!) so I turned to the dark side. The bubbly, brown side to be precise.

Ah, the sweet brown liquid that infamously had real cocaine in its original recipe, but is still just as dangerously addictive today. Coke has the most brilliant marketing slogan ever - "Coke adds Life". It gets right to the core of what everyone really wants – who doesn't want more "Life" in their life? Psychologically, it's brilliant in its simplicity, and I fell for it. I'd been exposed to all those Coke ads when I was younger, with gorgeous young things romping around on beaches, insinuating that Coke was the thing that made them so (and indeed "Coke Is It" was another of their brilliant slogans).

Of course, being out on the road and not confined to an office, I could indulge my new found Coke addiction pretty easily and without the guilt of co-workers watching my every move (is it just me, or do open-plan offices seem like a corporate version of Big Brother?) What made it worse, was that the warehouse had a vending machine with cans of coke for $2, when everywhere else was selling it for far more than that. I didn't even have to make small talk with someone behind a register to make the purchase. Just a little gold coin donation to the shiny, sparkling machine and it dispensed me another fix, no questions asked. Little wonder that I found it easy to down at least three or four cans a day, having to pop into the warehouse on a regular basis to pick up stock, samples or merchandising material. It was what sustained me through the day and I got rather grumpy if I didn't get my sugar hits at least several times a day. At the time, I blamed it on late nights, too much alcohol and fatigue from driving around all day, but it was simply the roller coaster effect of the sugar-high/crash cycle.

I was then approached to work for my next employer, a packaging manufacturer - supplier to the wine industry, as well as various beverage companies… including Coke. Oh dear. One of the "staff benefits" (are you starting to see a pattern here??) of this company was free access to the office fridges stocked with customers' products (non-alcoholic of course, they did have some semblance of responsibility towards their employees!) Fridges stacked high with Coke and, like the proverbial

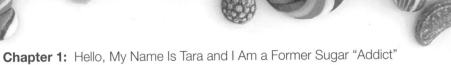

moth to the flame, I was drawn to those fridges, and the bottles seemed to just magically appear in my hand and down my throat.

This role also required me to spend a lot more time in the office that I was used to, due to the sheer amount of administration involved. Not only did this mean I was near those fridges many days of the week, I was also completely overexposed to the scourge that is the fundraising chocolate box. You know, the ones that every primary school sends home with kids to raise money. They're usually the purple company's brands and very cleverly priced at one or two dollars (nobody seems to notice that the chocolates weigh much, much less than the "same" ones at the Supermarket). There was always at least one co-worker raising money for their kids' school or another one topping up the sponsorship money for their fun-run. As soon as one box had been exhausted, there was always a back-up waiting to take its place. This constant availability, plus the fact that it again just required a little gold coin donation, often made completely anonymously, made it far too easy to feed my sugar addiction. This one had the added benefit of complete justification "but it's for charity!!"

So, my little sugar-demon was being well and truly fed. My sugar rush/ crash/rush cycle continued on and it seemed my model of the world had been set. Then, a couple of things happened. A "significant" birthday loomed, plus there was (yet another) restructure at work. I won't go into a huge amount of detail on that second point here, but perhaps I'll make that the subject of my next book! Suffice it to say, these things made me question what on earth I was doing with my life. I couldn't stay in such a negative environment and I got a real wake-up call that I was not following my heart, allowing other people to make decisions for me. My research and reading led me to discover a truly extraordinary system that changed my life completely and utterly – and I don't say that lightly.

After learning the techniques I'll be sharing with you in the following pages, I couldn't quite believe the difference in my outlook on life and, in particular, my attitude towards sugar.

After one particular seminar I returned to work on a Monday and, as was my habit, opened the office fridge and looked inside. That day was different though. That day I promptly closed it again without a second thought. Yes, it was THAT fridge – the one filled with Coke, the one I would take several bottles a day out of, and down them like they were water. I literally stopped in my tracks and stood still for a second or two, blinking like I'd just emerged into bright sunlight from a very dark cave. I felt like I'd just been struck by a bolt of lightning and my head was still buzzing from the electricity. What the $#@ had just happened to me? Years and years of addiction and habit had been erased, painlessly and with no effort on my part whatsoever!

Just to test things further, and to make sure I wasn't just having a Matrix-esque glitch, I stumbled towards the office kitchen. The permanently rotating box of fundraising chocolates sat on the bench, glinting purple under the fluorescent office lighting and begging for my loose change. Not a twitch or glimmer of desire emerged.

Nothing.

Nada.

Well, that was weird.

It just got stranger and stranger from that point – I turned down the generic office birthday cake every time it was offered to me, even if it was before lunch and I was starving. Things that I previously couldn't even contemplate without sugar, like black espresso coffee, became completely and utterly normal for me.

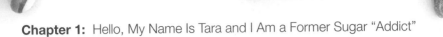

Since that fateful Monday, I've not touched Coke – it hasn't even tempted me in my previously favourite cocktail, a Cuba Libre. I just look at any fridge filled with brown liquid and my brain just says to me "That's not of interest" and moves on. Chocolate holds very little appeal, and on the rare occasion I buy a block of chocolate on sale (my bargain-hunter mentality is still very strong!) it can sit in the pantry for months. As for ice-cream? I eat it maybe twice a year now and never, ever for breakfast!

How did I do it? In a nutshell, I learned how to recognise and appreciate how my subconscious mind interacts with my conscious decision-making process. Once I understood how this worked, I figured out how I could make Outsmarting Sugar an unconscious habit, rather than something I had to use a great deal of Willpower or resolve to avoid.

I know you'll be pleasantly surprised by just how easy it is to incorporate these strategies into your daily life. That's what I love most about the system I've developed for you in this book – you can spend years and years in therapy, trying to use Willpower to stick to a diet or exercise regime or you can just use the techniques in this book and "flip the switch" instead!

Interested? I hope so! These skills are easy to learn and put into practice straight away. Read on to discover just how simple it is – but first, let's take a look at how we got into this mess in the first place.

CHAPTER 2

IT'S NOT YOUR FAULT!

"We have been brainwashed into craving a diet that is killing us. What we believe tastes good is generally what we have been socially conditioned to enjoy."

— Jane Velez-Mitchell

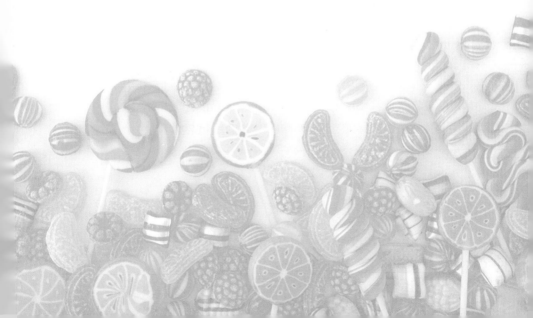

CHAPTER 2

IT'S NOT YOUR FAULT!

> *"Sugar is the fossil fuel of the food industry — cheap, acceptable, convenient and sold everywhere."*
> *— Tara Mitchell*

Although refined sugar has only been available for an extremely short period of time in human history, we are biologically pre-disposed to seek out sweetness as a reliable source of energy. Back when we had to chase lunch, coming across a clutch of berries, seasonal fruit or the syrupy goodness contained within a beehive was an amazing (if occasionally dangerous!) stroke of luck. Sweetness indicated that a food was high in energy and guaranteed it wasn't rotten or poisonous.

Before humans worked out how to cultivate plants and grow fruit trees, sweet-tasting foods were extremely rare in nature. So we became sweet-seeking missiles, ever ready to pounce upon this scarce source of energy whenever and wherever we could find it. For most of human history, consumption of sugar from any source at all was practically zero. Given the nomadic nature of ancient humans, storage was pretty much impossible. In fact, the first recorded evidence of dried fruit only dates back to 1,700 B.C. So we learned to gorge ourselves with any sweet substances we came across immediately and with gusto.

A Brief History of Refined Sugar

Clever humans first started to cultivate the wild sugarcane plant in New Guinea somewhere around 8,000 B.C. when it was simply cut and chewed to extract the sweet liquid inside. I'm not sure if you've ever tried to chew a piece of sugarcane, but they're extremely tough and getting any kind of sweetness from them is a pretty hard work-out. Back then, we had to put a great deal of effort into getting our sugar fix! From here, it spread throughout Southeast Asia and into India. Around 2,000 years ago Indians discovered how to crystallise sugarcane juice into what we now know as sugar. By extracting liquid from the cane through pounding or grinding, then boiling or drying in the sun, sand-like crystals were created which made transport a whole lot easier.

Seafaring traders then took these sweet granules to China and the Middle East. Right up until the Medieval period, sugar was so difficult and expensive to obtain, it was considered a 'fine spice' along with mace (nutmeg), ginger, cloves, and pepper. Only the wealthiest and most well-connected were able to purchase it. My, how times have changed!

Making its way to South America and the Caribbean in the mid-1500s, extraction was refined further. Due to the labour-intensive nature of growing and harvesting, plus the bulky nature of the canes, sugarcane production was highly localised. Plantations and mills started to pop up across the globe. By around 1500, technological improvements began turning it into a much cheaper bulk commodity, however a huge amount of labour was still needed. Our relentless desire for the sweet stuff is directly responsible for the slave trade in many parts of the world, which I find rather disturbing. We often think of sugar as just a sweet substance associated with innocent celebrations (like children's birthday parties), yet it has such a dark and socially divisive past.

In the 1700's, mechanisation of sugarcane processing meant sugar crystals could be produced cheaper than ever and, just like a viral online video, its popularity exploded beyond comprehension. In Great Britain for example, the consumption of sugar increased fivefold in the years between 1710 to 1770. The sugar tax was abolished in 1874, thereby making the sweet stuff affordable for the masses. Britain's health declined exponentially, with the rest of the world following suit.

Fast-forward to today, and sugarcane is the world's single largest crop. Sugar beet is the second largest source of sugar, providing us with about 30%. Since 1983, processed sugar consumption has been steadily increasing every year by around 28% and most Western countries consume up to 70 kilos per person per year. That's 16,800 teaspoons a year or 46 per day. Most health organisations recommend you should stay well under 9 a day!

So that's the condensed story of how sugar took over the world in a few short centuries. Contrast that period with the millennia of human history over which we were conditioned to believe that anything sweet is good – which it was, back when we had to undertake significant effort to find it. Now that processed sugar is so freely available, our challenge is to overcome generations of conditioning. Unfortunately, that conditioning is still happening and it's happening from the moment you're born.

Your Sugar Conditioning

The most frightening thing about your initial induction into sugar is there are no downsides whatsoever. In fact, as I'm sure you already know, the short-term associations with sugar are highly positive and even a fundamental part of human bonding. This isn't the case with other

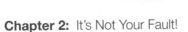
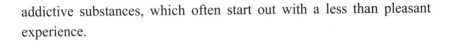

addictive substances, which often start out with a less than pleasant experience.

If you're not a smoker or an ex-smoker, you almost certainly know one. Every one of them has made the bold claim that they can "quit any time!" We hear this so often from smokers, it's become a cliché and is often used jokingly to deflect from an accusation of any kind of "addiction". This false sense of confidence actually explains why many people find it hard to give up sugar. I'll let you in on the secret, which has two parts:

PART ONE:

First, because the initial experience was so revolting, smokers don't even imagine it's addictive the first time they try it. Ask any smoker about the very first time they lit up – I'm willing to bet they'll tell you it was disgusting, they coughed their guts up and may even have thrown up! Thankfully for me, I found just being around smokers so repellent that I never took up the habit. But they kept at it, initially not because they liked it, but because it meant they were part of the "cool gang".

Some heroin addicts talk about being terrified of needles prior to their addiction and having to push through their fear to even try it for the first time. Again, overcoming something so horrendous leads to a false sense of being in control and a belief they can give up any time they want. There is still a small corner of their brain that remembers how repulsive their first time was and the effort that went into suppressing the horror of injecting themselves.

Even a drug as socially acceptable as alcohol is often an unpleasant experience (unless your first drink is sweet dessert wine or port as mine was, but that's a story for another day!). The first taste is pretty disgusting, especially to a younger palate tuned into sweetness. Beer and wine are quite bitter by their nature, so the taste is acquired over time and repeated exposure.

Not so with sugar – it's instantly appealing and our brain reasons "if it tastes good, it must be good for me!" Not only do you have millennia of human evolution to contend with, you've been trained from birth that sweetness is good and will fix all your troubles. Don't believe me? Just think about this…

Sugar Baby

From the moment you're born, you're trained that sweet-tasting things are comforting and soothing. Breast milk contains sugars, called oligosaccharides, as well as lactose, which is sweet-tasting. Babies have no other means of communication other than crying, and any form of discomfort, regardless of origin, is often met with an offer of milk. Even if you weren't actually hungry, the milk usually comes with mum's enveloping arms and lots of cuddles. This obviously creates an extremely powerful and primal association of sweetness with love and comfort. The ability of this magical sweet-tasting liquid to soothe you is falsely attributed by your developing brain – it was actually the cuddles you really wanted all along!

You might have had some chance of being able to outgrow this initial connection, if it weren't for our subsequent Western habits. Many of us are then put onto formula, which used to contain high levels of sugar (now banned in Australia) however it is still legal in many other countries around the world. Regardless of whether there's any added sugar in the formula, the high level of lactose from cow or goat's milk makes it taste sweet and cements our association with sweetness and someone caring for our needs.

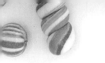

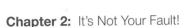

What a Sweet Kid!

Next, we're put onto solids and most of these are bought from the Supermarket. The bestselling ones contain apple, pear, banana, pumpkin, carrot and sweetcorn – the sweeter-tasting fruits and vegetables. Even "green vegetable" or the distinctly savoury-sounding "chicken, vegetables and quinoa" baby foods contain a percentage of apple or pear to make it more palatable for babies and toddlers.

Breakfast cereal designed for kids is sinfully high in sugar and often has fun, brightly-coloured animal mascots to increase the "kid appeal". We are often told that breakfast is the most important meal of the day, but if we're starting our kids' day with a high-sugar cereal, what sort of reinforcement does that create between sugar and an "important" meal?

Food Manufacturers have not only cornered the "kid appeal" market with breakfast cereal, they've also perfected the creation of the "time-poor" parent illusion. And isn't it wonderful that these multinational companies are looking after you, Mum & Dad, by providing such an array of "healthy" convenience foods to pack in the kids' lunch boxes? (You may or may not have picked up on my sarcasm there!!) The more obvious high-sugar products like choc-chip muesli bars are easy to spot, but what about noodle-snacks, boxes of raisins and white-bread sandwiches? The "after-school snack" market is also filled with novelty convenience foods, designed to keep kids occupied and "energised" (read: sugar-hyped!) for sports and other activities before dinner.

Juice often accompanies that sugary cereal for breakfast and the sugar-laden lunch or after-school snack. It's seen as "healthy and natural" because it's derived from fruit – which is good for us, right? Believe it or not, many juices contain more sugar per glass than soft drink! This makes them even more dangerous because we're not on guard when consuming them or giving them to our kids. It takes at least three or four apples to make a glass of juice. Have you ever tried to eat three or four apples in one sitting? Even two? It's almost impossible, even if you're really, really hungry! There's a reason Mother Nature wrapped up all that sugar with plenty of fibre and other nutrients – it slows down the rate at which the sugar enters your bloodstream and allows the energy to last much longer.

Then, the real fun begins! Birthday parties are debauched excesses of sugar, lollies, ice-cream and sugary soft drink. Most people's immediate reaction to a small child at a birthday party running around like a headless chicken is "Oh dear - someone's had too much red cordial, haven't they?!", with a sense of endearment. It's seen as OK because they're not doing it that often… but they're being set up for a lifetime of associating sweet things with celebration and fun. Try to imagine fairs and carnivals without fairy-floss, toffee-apples and hot cinnamon doughnuts. Easter without chocolate eggs. Christmas without candy canes, gingerbread men and chocolate Advent calendars. Australia Day without lamingtons. Halloween without candy corn. The link between sugar and celebration, fun or holidays is really quite scary when you think about it.

All Grown Up?

Once you've graduated past the minefield of sugary processed foods aimed at kids and specifically designed to create an intense relationship with a brand, you finally grow up and get to choose your own food – hooray!! Or do you?? You're now subject to a whole new set of advertising and brainwashing. You're now working full time, or perhaps attending some kind of further education. Cereal still takes pride of

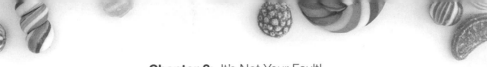

place at the breakfast table, but don't be fooled into thinking the 'adult' versions contain any less sugar.

Now your "healthy" cereal options are joined by muffins, exotic additions to your juice like pineapple and guava, as well as pastries, low-fat yoghurt and fruit breads. You can now guzzle soft drink with reckless abandon in defiance of all the times your intake was limited as a child. But now there are also "sports drinks" (more often used as hangover cures than for actual sports!) and all kinds of designer energy drinks vying for your attention. Cakes, doughnuts and chocolate form an integral part of your workplace bonding rituals, and you couldn't even imagine dinner without dessert. Is it any wonder we don't think we have a real problem when sugar is such an integral part of the entire human experience in the Western world?

PART TWO:

Now, I think you get the first part of the reason that sugar is so hard to "quit" – modern sugar conditioning is very real and almost seems innocent in its attachment to fun and convenience. The second part of the secret is that sugar has a very insidious effect on your mood and overall health. We don't sit up and take notice of its effects until it's too late. You're probably aware of some of the long-term effects of a high sugar diet, given the media coverage in recent years (if you haven't been paying attention, I'll cover this in the next chapter – What Sugar Really Does to Your Body) but for now, think about the effects of sugar versus alcohol as an example.

Punch Drunk

Getting drunk has a fairly immediate effect – you often feel more chatty and perhaps a little bit invincible, then gradually more and more tipsy and befuddled. Many people say it loosens their inhibitions, making them to say or do things that they wouldn't. Some people unfortunately get violent. You can see the effects of excessive consumption on any given Saturday night after dark in the city. You may have even felt them yourself and had to deal with the aftermath of a hangover the next day. The thought of another drink turns your stomach. You know that too much is bad for you, there are government campaigns against overindulgence, the word "alcoholic" implies someone who's truly dependent on it, and is taken quite seriously. There are clinics and drying-out camps, interventions and entire charity campaigns focussed on quitting alcohol such as "Dry July", "Dryalthon" and "OcSober". These are all very worthy causes, and help to raise much-needed money for charities that do some amazing work for those who really need our help. Alcohol's immediacy of effect makes you sit up and take notice of what you're consuming and really think about it next time you're offered a drink.

But excess sugar consumption? Its effects aren't often felt until years later. You might get a quick surge of energy, but it doesn't take long for the sugar rush to wear off. Some people speak of a sugar "hangover" if they've over-indulged, but they're happy to eat or drink more sugar-laden food and drink hours – sometimes even minutes – later. A self-confessed "chocoholic" is seen as cute and adorable, and it's only when it gets to morbid obesity or other extremes of health issues that it's taken seriously. Can you imagine "Chocolate-free December" (maybe we should rename it "Diabetes December"!) as a charity event? Many charities actually have chocolate boxes as fundraisers and of course the Girl Guide biscuit drives are world famous. Sugar is in so many

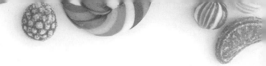

processed foods that it's nigh on impossible to isolate a single food or drink to give up and raise money for. It's added to all sorts of savoury foods – tomato sauce, pasta sauce, baked beans, soy sauce, mayonnaise, bread, ready-made soups and I've even found it listed as an ingredient in a jar of crushed garlic!

Because sugar is so ingrained in our diet, we barely notice the effect of it on our physiology. I know I've definitely felt the effects of too much coffee (racing heartbeat, grinding teeth and shaking hands anyone?) but, whilst I might have felt a bit ill and annoyed at having to scrape the fuzz off my teeth after chowing down on too much sugar, the immediate reaction is nowhere near as obvious.

After reading all of this, you probably realise that, up until now, you may not have been consciously aware of exactly how much you've been conditioned to be attracted to sugar. But is it really all that bad, you might ask? The fact that you've picked up this book makes me think that you know sugar isn't that great for you.

Just in case you had any doubts, read on to discover just what sugar does to your body and why you should be afraid… very afraid.

CHAPTER 3

WHAT SUGAR REALLY DOES TO YOU AND WHY YOU SHOULD BE AFRAID, VERY AFRAID

"Sugar is the next tobacco, without a doubt, and that industry should be scared. It should be taxed just like tobacco and anything else that can, frankly, destroy lives."

— Jamie Oliver

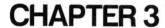

CHAPTER 3

WHAT SUGAR REALLY DOES TO YOU AND WHY YOU SHOULD BE AFRAID, VERY AFRAID

> *"The real cost of processed sugar is not your grocery bill, but your doctor's bill."*
> — Tara Mitchell

Processed sugar contains no vital nutrients. None. At all. No proteins, essential fats, vitamins or minerals. There's absolutely nothing there that your body needs to survive.

Now, when we're talking about sugar, not only are we talking about the white, extracted, processed stuff that sits in your sugar bowl (that you're now about to stop adding to your tea and coffee!) but also the hidden sugars in just about every packaged food and drink on Supermarket shelves. What we're *not* talking about is whole fruit – it's impossible to overdo it on fruit, because the sugars are neatly packaged up with fibre and nutrients.

But exactly how much is too much? Remember, most health authorities recommend:

- No more than 24 grams, or 6 teaspoons of sugar, per day for women

- No more than 36 grams, or 9 teaspoons of sugar, per day for men

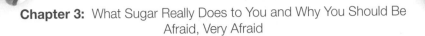

For reference, a single 375mL can of regular Coca-Cola has *39 grams* of sugar!

Adults have five litres of blood circulating and about two teaspoons of glucose should be present at any one time. One Coke raises the blood sugar to five times its normal level, for at least four hours. My Coke habit alone saw me ingesting at least 117 grams of sugar *every day* - and that was on top of my "healthy" breakfast smoothie, muesli bars, chocolate, lollies, sauces, dressings, dips and various other packaged food throughout the day.

What does your daily intake look like? Check the labels of your food, count the teaspoons you're stirring into your tea and coffee and calculate your total:

Breakfast _____

Morning Tea _____

Lunch _____

Afternoon Tea _____

Dinner _____

After Dinner _____

TOTAL _____

When we constantly overload our system with too much glucose, and especially fructose, all sorts of health problems arise. Many are well documented, but some we're just starting to learn about now. Like what? Well, here are just a few of the things excess sugar does…

Sugar Triggers Inflammation

You know how your ankle puffs up like a balloon when you sprain it? That's inflammation at work. Its job is to deal with cell injury and initiate tissue repair, which you see and feel as pain, heat, redness and swelling. Bombarding your body with excess sugar makes it think it's under attack and it responds accordingly. Chronic inflammation affects every aspect of your health and is directly linked to a whole host of serious diseases, including atherosclerosis, rheumatoid arthritis and cancer.

It's also the source of a whole host of other more 'minor' ailments, as well as your garden-variety aches and pains. What I thought was years of skiing catching up with my knees was actually inflammation from years of too much sugar catching up with me. I even resorted to cortisone injections to relieve the pain and swelling, but they couldn't help me, where Outsmarting Sugar has.

Sugar Causes Insulin Resistance and Diabetes

Insulin resistance is the precursor to Type-2 Diabetes, one of the fastest rising chronic diseases in the world. I'm sure you've heard of insulin and know it's really important, but this isn't a biology textbook so we'll keep it simple. Basically, insulin shifts glucose out of your bloodstream by 'opening the door' into your cells and telling them to prioritise burning glucose for energy instead of fat. Consuming too much sugar means your body needs more and more insulin to keep up, just like a junkie needs higher and higher doses to achieve the same high.

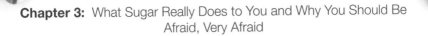

Insulin resistance means the cell doors get stuck and they don't open properly. When this happens, your cells can't let all the glucose in, leaving it to build up in your bloodstream. This triggers the pancreas to make more insulin, which doesn't help because the cell doors are still stuck, so your blood glucose levels keep rising, which triggers the pancreas to make more insulin… and around and around we go! Eventually, the pancreas just can't keep up and blood glucose rises to dangerous levels, which is at the point where Type-2 Diabetes occurs. You'll need daily injections of insulin to control your blood glucose, which I think is pretty scary, don't you? If injections don't bother you too much, perhaps some of these nasty complications might:

- **Heart Disease and Stroke.** The glucose molecule is quite rough (think of a granulated sugar crystal) and blood vessels aren't designed to transport huge numbers of them. The jagged edges nick the walls, causing damage. Your body provides its own band-aids in the form of low-density lipoprotein (LDL) cholesterol, which has been labelled the "bad" cholesterol. More damage means more LDL is needed to patch up those walls, which can end up restricting blood flow and leads to heart disease. Some of the patches detach themselves from the walls, travelling through your system until they lodge in a smaller vessel and completely block it – you know this as a stroke. Sugar has literally gotten away with murder for years – cholesterol was framed!

- **Neuropathy.** Glucose molecules also damage your nerves, leading to permanent numbness in your extremities. That doesn't sound too bad, until you think about the fact that you can injure yourself quite badly and not even notice. The digestive nervous system can also be compromised, which means your stomach doesn't work properly. I'll leave that one to your imagination…

- **Amputation.** If you've developed neuropathy and hurt yourself, the news only gets worse. Because you're also likely to have very poor circulation, wounds often fail to heal and can go gangrenous, meaning you might lose a limb. I don't know about you, but I'm very attached to mine and would much rather keep them that way!

- **Blindness.** The tiny, defenceless blood vessels behind the eye can easily be roughed up by a gang of glucose molecules, causing them to bulge, swell and leak blood. Left untreated, blindness will result. Globally, diabetes is the number one cause of blindness in people under 75 and is almost completely preventable. So it turns out there's more than one sin that can make you go blind…

- **Kidney Failure.** Your poor old kidneys try to take up where the pancreas failed to rid your body of excess glucose. They work triple shifts with no tea breaks, trying to flush it all out. Just like a human working three jobs to try and make ends meet, they get overworked and eventually collapse from sheer exhaustion. You'll need to be hooked in to a dialysis machine for several hours a day to sub in for their shifts, which can really interfere with your social life.

Sugar Keeps You Up at Night (and not in a good way…)

Your sugar rush-crash-rush daily cycle sets you up for a bad night's sleep, which then feeds the next day's cycle. Have you ever woken up exhausted and your immediate reaction is to brew yourself a tea or coffee loaded with sugar? Congratulations – you've just jump-started the cycle again! When your blood's swamped with glucose, the hormone cortisol (also known as the "stress hormone") is released, which is what gets you the sugar-rush you've been chasing. Guess what? Cortisol released at the wrong time of day causes major disruption to your ability to sleep.

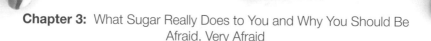

Reckon you can be smart and time your sugar-crash just before you hit the hay? Good luck with that one. Your body then releases more hormones to regulate low glucose levels back to normal. Those hormones also stimulate brain activity, which makes for broken sleep and some even say it contributes to nightmares.

Sugar Messes with Your Immune System

Ironically, a depressed immune system caused by eating too much sugar can leave you feeling low in energy. Like me, you might have been conditioned to believe that energy can only be boosted with a sugar hit, so it sets up yet another vicious cycle! A strong immune system means you can fight off most things thrown at you. Have you ever noticed how you tend to pick up every bug going around when you're feeling a bit sluggish? You may also notice that your body will not heal cuts and wounds as quickly.

This was a massive one for me: I would be struck down with every cold or flu that happened to be doing the rounds, which led to a chronic cough that wouldn't budge for months. I blamed it on office air-conditioning drying out my throat.

I also used to get debilitating hay fever every spring and I dreaded even venturing outside without being dosed up to the eyeballs with antihistamines – which, of course, cause drowsiness, which I then tried to fix with more sugar! Since Outsmarting Sugar, I rarely get sick and "hay fever season" scares me about as much as a wet paper bag!

Sugar Gives You a Kick in the Teeth

Everyone knows that sugar is bad for your teeth. How many times were you told as a kid that too many sweets will "rot your teeth"? It wasn't just mum trying to prevent you going hyper from too much red cordial, the link between sugar and tooth decay has been well researched and established for many decades.

Soft drinks are the worst of all for your teeth – not only do they contain vast amounts of sugar, they are highly acidic and will literally dissolve tooth enamel. To refresh your high-school chemistry, the pH scale ranges from 1 (most acidic) to 14 (least acidic). The pH of soft drinks can be as low as 2.4 – for comparison, battery acid is 1!! The damage done to your teeth by soft drinks is as bad as, and sometimes even worse than, long-term drug use. Yikes!

Sugar Steals Your Bones

Remember how I justified my ice-cream and low-fat milk intake by thinking it would prevent the osteoporosis my grandmother suffered from? Turns out I was actually doing myself more harm than good. High blood sugar causes calcium to be excreted through your urine, so your body never gets a chance to use it. Plus, the high acidity of soft drinks actually leaches calcium and other minerals from your bones, which can cause them to become even more brittle over time. To complete the trifecta - the excess cortisol that keeps you up at night is also bad for your bones. Oh dear…

Sugar Wrecks Your Skin

You probably know there's a huge anti-ageing market with companies making several billion dollars a year from our desire to defy nature. Although spokesmodels will try and convince you otherwise, you can't stop or reverse ageing, but you can certainly accelerate it by eating too much sugar! Collagen and elastin are proteins that help keep your

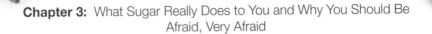

skin looking supple and youthful, but fructose and glucose molecules are having none of that, and like to attach themselves to these proteins uninvited. Kinda like that weird guy nobody knows at your house party. This process is called glycation and it makes things brittle and stiff, causing skin to look dry, dull and older. As well as ageing your skin, too much sugar has been found to aggravate other skin conditions, like acne, rosacea and eczema.

Sugar Feeds The Enemy

It's not called "The Big C" for nothing – cancer is one of the leading causes of death worldwide and is characterised by exponential multiplication of cells. Insulin is a key hormone in regulating cell growth and, as we know, excess sugar consumption really messes with your insulin production. There's still some controversy around whether sugar actually "feeds" cancer specifically (all of your cells use glucose for energy) but the fact that processed sugar impacts on known cancer indicators like obesity, inflammation, insulin sensitivity, immunity and high acidity levels should give you cause for concern.

Sugar also feeds the gut flora which can throw your digestive system out of balance, contributing to gas, bloating and constipation, as well as more persistent conditions like irritable bowel syndrome (IBS) and chronic fatigue syndrome. Let's just say that for me, things are moving a lot more freely since I Outsmarted Sugar!

Sugar Makes You Fat in Sneaky Ways

Sugar is just like a ninja assassin when it comes to weight gain – it's the ones you never see coming that you need to be most afraid of. Sure, we all know cake and ice-cream are not your waistline's friends, but they're

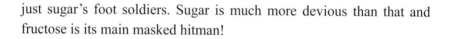

just sugar's foot soldiers. Sugar is much more devious than that and fructose is its main masked hitman!

Fructose makes up 50% of processed sugar and up to 90% in 'safe' sweeteners like agave syrup. Unlike every other food molecule (even glucose) fructose doesn't flip the satiety, or the "I'm full, stop eating now!", switch in your brain. This is a relic from our ancestors, when fructose was a rare and special treat, only found packaged up in whole fruit. Back then, it was a great idea to eat as much as possible of this scarce energy source. Now that fructose doesn't always bring its friends with benefits i.e. the nutrients and fibre in fruit found in fruit, it's far too easy to overeat without gettin' no satisfaction.

Fructose also increases the hormone ghrelin, which fuels hunger – making you feel hungry, even when you know you're full. This effect occurs even if you just look at something sweet, as your brain is so well-trained to respond to fructose. Now you know why it's easy to drink a huge amount of calories in a cola with your burger meal, and why, when you can't eat two burgers, you still have room for dessert. There really is an extra "dessert stomach", but it's in your brain – not your belly!

Because sugar messes with your sleep patterns, you may have found it difficult to get off that hamster wheel of using sugar to boost the energy you've lost from lack of sleep that sugar caused in the first place. By constantly stoking your fire with sugar, your body gets used to burning sugar, not fat and that fat will start accumulating.

Much worse than not fitting into your favourite jeans, fat gathers internally around your liver (especially when you consume high levels of fructose, which can only be metabolised in the liver) causing NAFLD. No, that's not the latest Top-40 boy-band, it's the acronym for Non-

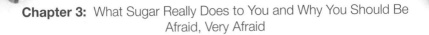

alcoholic Fatty Liver Disease. You could end up with cirrhosis of the liver or even liver cancer.

Sugar Messes with Your Mental Health

What sugar does to your body is scary enough, but what's even more frightening is what it can do to your mind. Research suggests that the sugar high-crash-high roller coaster may have a massive impact on our mental health. You might think that giant tub of ice-cream is going to make you feel better (and it might, for a second or two!) but the total opposite is likely to be true longer-term.

Your brain can be quite easily tricked by bio-feedback – that is, it assumes you are feeling a certain emotion based on physical cues. This is why simply smiling can make you feel better: your brain knows you only smile when you're happy, therefore you must be happy! Think of all the bio-feedback caused by the sugar-rush-crash cycle:

SUGAR RUSH

EFFECTS ON BODY:	BRAIN'S INTERPRETATION:
Elevated heart rate	I am excited!
Cortisol rush	I am energetic!!
Adrenaline rush	I am wide awake!!
High blood glucose	I am friendly!!
Dopamine release	I am loved!!
Serotonin release	I am high!!

SUGAR CRASH

EFFECTS ON BODY	BRAIN'S INTERPRETATION:
Low blood sugar	I am depressed
Lethargic	I am sad
Brain fog	I am anxious
Fatigued	I am tired
Shaky	I am panicky
Tense	I am stressed
Blurred Vision	I am paranoid
Excess Cortisol	I am scared
Excess Adrenaline	I am primed and ready for fight or flight

No wonder there's a strong link between high sugar consumption and the risk of depression! The momentary boost in mood from sugar just isn't worth it, especially if you are already in poor mental health. Short Term Gain. Long Term Pain.

Alzheimer's disease and dementia have long been considered hereditary disorders and an inevitable part of ageing. Mounting evidence suggests otherwise, with studies showing that Alzheimer's patients brains have been impaired by insulin resistance (sound familiar?) and are unable to use glucose to produce energy properly. It's now at the point where the medical community refer to Alzheimer's as Type-3 diabetes. You're also twice as likely to develop Alzheimer's or another form of dementia if you already have Type-2 diabetes.

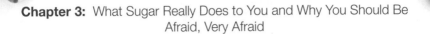

Even if you don't develop a serious mental condition, processed sugar is not your brain's friend. Insulin resistance, inflammation and interference with proteins can also disrupt communication between the brain cells responsible for learning, memory formation and higher thinking. At the very least, sugar will make you dumber and more forgetful!

Can I Improve My Health by Outsmarting Sugar?

The human 'body and mind' interaction is a complex synergy but, just like when you drive a car or a computer, you don't need to be an IT specialist or mechanic to know when things are going wrong! If you suffer from any of the following (or if you have a family history of them), Outsmarting Sugar will definitely have benefits for you.

Tick the ones that affect you or your family to find out exactly how many areas you could improve:

_____ Acne	_____ Irritable Bowel Syndrome
_____ Rosacea	_____ Premature Ageing
_____ ADHD	_____ Obesity
_____ Fatty Liver Disease	_____ Depression
_____ Diabetes	_____ Insulin Resistance
_____ Hashimoto's Disease	_____ Mood Swings
_____ Hypoglycaemia	_____ Kidney Stones
_____ Candida	_____ Constipation
_____ Dementia	_____ Alzheimer's Disease
_____ Tooth Decay	_____ Insomnia

_____ Inflammation of Joints   _____Heart Disease

_____Stroke   _____Vision Problems

_____Chronic Fatigue   _____Anxiety

_____Cancer   _____Thyroid Problems

_____Gum Disease   _____Hay Fever

_____Osteoporosis   _____High Cholesterol

_____Constant Colds and Coughs   _____Gas and Bloating

CHAPTER 4

WHO'S REALLY IN CHARGE OF YOUR BRAIN?

"Addiction isn't about substance — you aren't addicted to the substance, you are addicted to the alteration of mood that the substance brings."

— Susan Cheever

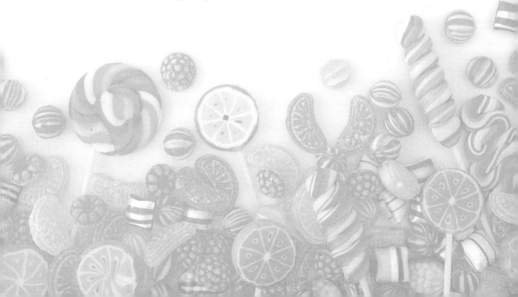

CHAPTER 4

WHO'S REALLY IN CHARGE OF YOUR BRAIN?

"Saying we only use 10% of our brains is like saying traffic lights only use 33% of their capacity!"
— Tara Mitchell

Do you really have an "addiction" to sugar? There's plenty of clinical studies that suggest it's possible, demonstrating that sugar activates your brain in the same regions as drugs like cocaine and morphine. It's also true that sugar can cause a release of dopamine, serotonin and beta-endorphin (a.k.a. the 'feel-good' hormones) in the brain, and by much more than our ancestors were ever exposed to in foods found in nature. These hormones improve our mood, raise our self-esteem and reduce our anxiety – who wouldn't want more of that? Thus our sugar-seeking missile is launched, and we seek out this high again and again. In fact, we train ourselves so well that a study found simply showing a picture of a milkshake to sugar "addicts" activated the same reward centres of the brain as actually consuming it. No wonder visual advertising is so effective!

There are also a myriad of trials and experiments that show rats prefer sugar over cocaine, even when they've been conditioned to be addicted to cocaine. Rodents share some similar characteristics as humans (did you know mice love sugar almost as much as humans do?) which is why they're unfortunately used for lab testing, but they lack the highly complex emotions that are the real source of human sugar "addiction".

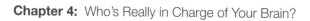
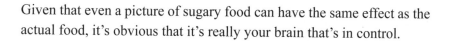

Given that even a picture of sugary food can have the same effect as the actual food, it's obvious that it's really your brain that's in control.

We still really don't understand much about how the brain works and even now, there are still a lot of myths out there. Have you heard of the saying "Humans only use 10% of their brain capacity?" It's been falsely attributed to many, the most famous being Albert Einstein, however it's really just an urban myth. It's one of those sayings that we now seem to accept as being true just because it's been repeated so often – sort of like:

"Have a break, have a Kit Kat", or

"A Mars a day helps you work, rest and play", or

"Coke is Life!"

The 10% thing dates back to the early 19th century, when we knew even less about the inner workings of the human brain. In reality, saying humans only use 10% of our brain is like saying traffic lights only use 33% of their capacity!

You see, just like traffic lights, each part of our brain is designed for a specific use. There are many activities that your brain needs to control, ranging from thoughts, reactions and behaviours, as well as the physical human mechanics like breathing, blood circulation and digesting food. It's best that these are split into different areas, so you can keep functioning if one part gets damaged.

Generally speaking, it all works pretty well together and usually without you even being consciously aware of it. There are three levels of functions controlled by your brain:

1) Unconscious – things like your blood circulation, that you don't have any conscious control over.

2) Semi-conscious – your breathing for example. You usually don't think too much about this, but once you become aware of it, you can choose how to breathe, but not stop it entirely.

3) Conscious – you have complete control of these functions, which include your emotions and how you react to external events. You actually choose whether the best response is to finish that tub of ice-cream or not, although it may not feel like it sometimes!

The reason this control escapes you on occasion is that the different parts of our brain have competing interests and can actually work against your conscious mind. But please don't get mad at your brain – it's just trying to protect you!

Why on earth would part of your brain actively try and contradict your conscious behaviour? Think of it as the over-protective parent that really does want the best for you, but is a little old-fashioned and can seriously cramp your style! The part of the brain that does this is called the Amygdala and it's the most primal and ancient section. So much so, that it's often called your "Lizard Brain", as its impulsive reactions to external forces are pretty much the same as those any reptile trying to protect itself! The Amygdala is quite short-sighted and impulsive. Its main mission in life is to keep you safe from the sabre-toothed tiger – beyond that, it doesn't really know or care what happens next.

You can see from the diagram below that the Amygdala is at the very core of your brain and the other parts (that control perception and higher mental functions) have grown around it as humans have evolved.

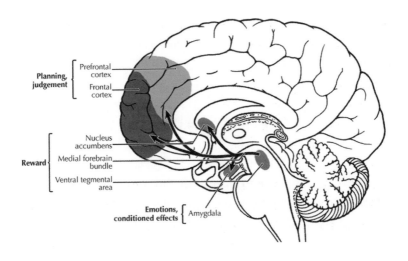

[The Brain with Amygdala]

The Amygdala is concerned with the most basic function of all – keeping you safe from harm. Now, despite its best intentions, the way it does this doesn't always marry up with what you think of as "safe" in this modern world. Let's go back to lunch-chasing days, when humans lived in tribes and "safety in numbers" wasn't just a catchphrase, it was a life-or-death situation.

If, for whatever reason, you were rejected from the tribe and left to fend for yourself, it's likely you wouldn't last long on your own. Even if you were a very skilled hunter or gatherer, the isolation from human support and assistance in case you fell ill or were injured, meant you would probably die quite quickly. If exposure to the elements didn't get you, there were always wild animals around that would happily make you dinner! The Amygdala can be accused of many things, but being a slow learner is definitely not one of them. It's lightning-fast at making connections that help you in split-second, life-saving decisions, and that's why it's in charge of your "Fight or Flight" response.

The Number One mission for the Amygdala is to save you from dying and it lives by the equation:

Rejection = Death

It will do everything it can to ensure you "fit in" and keep your place in your tribe. If it sees you doing something that might get you "rejected", it will react very quickly to counter it. Conversely, if it works out there's something you can do to be accepted, it will propel you towards this action. You may have been aware of this in high school, when you did or wore all kinds of strange things and put it down to "peer pressure". Despite many teenagers displaying tendencies to the contrary, the one thing a human will go to huge lengths to avoid is death!

So, now you know who's really in charge of your brain, what's the Amygdala's role in your sugar "addiction"?

There's no denying sugar's seductive power, especially when it comes packaged up as a solution to emotionally charged events like a break-up or highly-stressful day at work. Whilst sugar can seem like the answer in the moment, the side effects will catch up with you eventually – and you already know why you should be very afraid of these! After a while, scoffing sugar causes more problems than benefits and, what's worse, it hasn't actually killed any of those negative emotions you've been trying to suppress.

Simply using Willpower to deprive yourself of sugar won't help either – this will just leave you feeling even more sad and hard done by, because

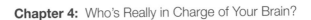

you can't have what you think you really want. In seeking a fix for this sadness, your well-trained brain will eventually lead you right back to – you guessed it – sugar! The Amygdala is lurking around here and loves to jump in and help the only way it knows how.

When you're "rejected", either by a lover or your boss, the lizard brain is worried you'll "die" and so goes into survival mode by – yep, you guessed it again – scoffing sugar. Because it's still thinking the way it was trained prehistorically, it thinks you need lots of energy to cope on your own without the help of your tribe. Remember, you'll need to build a shelter, hunt and gather whatever food you can, as well as protect yourself from wild animals (and possibly wild humans!), so you'll need all your strength. Plus, the Amygdala knows that you'll get a rush of those feel-good hormones from sugar that you'd normally get from human interaction. See, it really does have your best interests at heart! This strengthens your emotional dependence on sugar each and every time you reach for a chocolate instead of a hug.

Ah, emotions - some might say they're the true hallmark of humanity, others say they're the cause of all our troubles! Emotions are triggered by a complex set of associations and they can be totally different for every single one of us. Fear is a classic example of this complexity in humans. Did you know that when we're born, we only have two fears:

1) Loud noises

2) Being dropped

Makes sense when you're a freshly-minted human – loud noises probably meant something like a sabre-tooth tiger growl, another human screaming or a thunder clap. Being dropped meant well, you know…

Then think about all the fears and neuroses that develop once we become adults. Some of them are fairly common and seem completely understandable to me, like:

- Arachnophobia. Fear of spiders. Yep, I get that. No questions.

- Ophidiophobia. Fear of snakes. Makes total sense to me.

- Apiphobia. Fear of bees. Personally, I'm OK with them, however for some people they are literally killers.

But some of our modern fears seem completely ridiculous if you think about them:

- Paraskevidekatriaphobia. Fear of Friday the 13th. Really. Apparently 8% of Americans have this phobia. I'm not sure if this says more about superstitions or Hollywood movie producers!

- Cacomorphobia. Fear of fat people. What. The??

- Kinemortophobia. Fear of zombies. This is my personal favourite. Humans are so irrational we've managed to create a phobia for a totally imaginary creature!

And then there are others that are shared by almost all of us, but have no basis in common sense. Like the fear of public speaking. The majority of people are more terrified of standing up and speaking in front of a group than the Grim Reaper himself. Yet when you think about it, we all talk out loud to an audience every day – even if sometimes it's just the cat! Honestly, when most people are watching a speaker, they're more

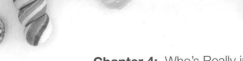
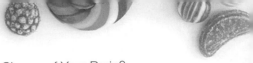

likely to be thinking "Thank goodness it's not me up there!" than paying attention to whether you've used the correct syntax in your sentence structure.

The common denominator in all of these is our old friend the Amygdala, trying to keep us safe. Yes indeed, even the fear of public speaking can be traced back to the Lizard Brain. It's worried that you'll say something wrong or look silly in front of the "tribe" and therefore be rejected. What's interesting about human emotions is that they're completely manufactured by our own individual brains. Let me give you a personal example of this (and I'm sure you can think of your own):

If I come face-to-face with a German Shepherd dog, I am immediately frozen to the spot with fear. I will back away slowly and carefully and wouldn't dream of approaching such a fearsome animal. It could be the most loving, well-trained, "man's best friend" on the planet, but I would still be completely terrified.

Yet if my partner Toby were to be faced with the very same animal, he would rush forward open-armed, squealing with joy to give the dog a massive cuddle!

The difference? I'm very wary of large dogs, German Shepherds in particular, after being chased down the street by a very aggressive one when I was six. Toby, on the other hand, had a beautiful pet Rottweiler-German Shepherd cross as a pet and feels nothing but love towards big dogs.

My Amygdala: Big Dog = Scary, run for your life!

Toby's Amygdala: Big Dog = Loving cuddle monster

What's this got to do with sugar "addiction"? Well, I'm a very strong believer that what we have simply named "addiction" is actually far more complex than that. The huge number of subtle influences you're exposed to over your lifetime create a web of entanglement and it can be pretty hard to escape – unless you know how. This web traps you in a pattern of compulsive emotional attraction to sugar and it's almost like someone is pushing you to eat it.

Sound familiar? Try out this little test to see if you have a compulsive emotional attraction:

Read the following statements and circle the number indicating how much you agree or disagree with the statement.

(1)   (2)   (3)   (4)   (5)
Never   Rarely   Sometimes Often   Frequently

a)   I buy a family sized box/pack of chocolate/cookies/ice-cream with the intention of sharing it or eating just a little at a time. I then eat the whole lot in one sitting.

   (1)   (2)   (3)   (4)   (5)

b)   I feel weird if I watch a movie without ice-cream/chocolate/lollies.

   (1)   (2)   (3)   (4)   (5)

c)   Any time I am bored or tired, the first thing I reach for is something sugary.

   (1)   (2)   (3)   (4)   (5)

d) For me, eating chocolate/cake/cookies/ice-cream is a way of coping with stress.

    (1)   (2)   (3)   (4)   (5)

e) I feel that something inside pushed me to eat chocolate/cookies/ice-cream.

    (1)   (2)   (3)   (4)   (5)

f) I have a strong and uncontrollable urge to eat chocolate/cookies/ice-cream.

    (1)   (2)   (3)   (4)   (5)

g) I feel guilty after eating too much chocolate/cookies/ice-cream because it seemed unreasonable.

    (1)   (2)   (3)   (4)   (5)

h) I hide chocolate/cookies in my desk at work, or around my home so I don't have to share with others.

    (1)   (2)   (3)   (4)   (5)

i) As soon as I enter a Supermarket or other shop, I have an irresistible urge to head to the confectionery/cookie/ice-cream aisle.

    (1)   (2)   (3)   (4)   (5)

j) I think it is perfectly reasonable to eat a whole tub of ice-cream to cope with a romantic relationship breakup.

    (1)   (2)   (3)   (4)   (5)

k) I have felt sick after eating too much chocolate/cookies/ice-cream.

   (1)   (2)   (3)   (4)   (5)

l) I identify with the term "chocoholic" or feel that I am "addicted" to sugar

   (1)   (2)   (3)   (4)   (5)

m) I have thought "If I had to do it over again, I wouldn't have done that" and felt sorry for eating something sugary.

   (1)   (2)   (3)   (4)   (5)

Calculate your score:

Add up all the numbers that you circled to get your total score.

Write it down here:

——————

Score 13–25

You are Zen-like in your reaction to sugar. Nothing much fazes you but you occasionally let the Lizard Brain have what it wants after careful consideration.

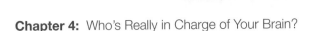

Score 26–32

You do pretty well when faced with sugary temptations, but you slip up sometimes. Overall, you should be pretty pleased with yourself, but you know you could do even better.

Score 33–41

You quite often let that Lizard Brain take control, even when your higher self knows better. You probably get a little disappointed and even a bit mad with yourself. You could really do with some help, but aren't quite sure how to get it. Read on!

Score 42 or more

Your Lizard Brain is in charge, at large and totally in control of your actions. You need to get that thing on a leash! But how??

I know it might seem like the world is stacked against you – as we saw in Chapter 2, you've been primed to be a sugar-seeking missile, not just within your own lifetime, but for generations before you. Plus, your Amygdala is a powerful force within you that will quite often steer you in the wrong direction (even if it's for the right reasons!).

If this is the case, then how come some people find it easy to control their sugar intake? They can have just a square or two of a family block of chocolate, they can take just one scoop of ice-cream from a tub and place it back in the freezer or they can take just one biscuit from a packet.

You now know some of it's about the complex web of interactions that have taken place throughout your entire life. You might think the rest of it is all about that amazing mythical creature called Willpower but, as you'll find out shortly, pure Willpower doesn't work long-term – but I'll show you what does!

CHAPTER 5

WHY WILLPOWER DOESN'T WORK... BUT I'LL SHOW YOU WHAT DOES

"Willpower is trying very hard not to do something you want to do very much."

— John Ortberg

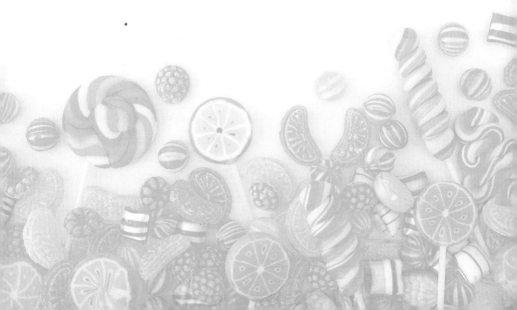

CHAPTER 5

WHY WILLPOWER DOESN'T WORK... BUT I'LL SHOW YOU WHAT DOES

"Save your Willpower for the important stuff — like staying out of jail!"
— Tara Mitchell

Ah, Willpower! We humans have granted it mythical Godlike status and view those who have appeared to master it as Gods themselves. Every single survey undertaken as to why we don't exercise more, eat better or save more money for retirement puts "Lack of Willpower" at Number One. It appears that "Lack of Willpower" is the single biggest barrier for us poor little humans!

So how would you rate yours? Take this quick quiz to find out – circle the answer that represents you best (be honest!):

1) Your friend gives you a present a month before your birthday and tells you not to open it until your actual birthday. You:

    a)   Open it the second they leave.

    b)   Shake it, inspect it, analyse and agonise over it until your birthday.

    c)   Leave it alone until your birthday. The surprise is so much sweeter that way.

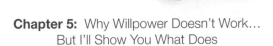

2) If you promise yourself to stop at one chocolate biscuit, you:

    a)   Stop at one chocolate biscuit. Then immediately eat the rest of the packet.

    b)   Stop at two or three chocolate biscuits.

    c)   Stop at one chocolate biscuit, if you have one at all.

3) You get $500 cash unexpectedly (yay!) You:

    a)   Spend all of it immediately.

    b)   Try to stretch it as long as you can, and have a bit leftover.

    c)   Bank all of it. That interest adds up!

4) If you resolve to get up an hour early, can you do it?

    a)   Not unless your life depended on it.

    b)   You can get up earlier, but you'll hit the snooze button a couple of times.

    c)   You can definitely do it. In fact, you don't even need to set the alarm earlier!

5) How would you describe your exercise habits?

    a)   You don't exercise.

    b)   You exercise here and there, but not as much as you know you should.

    c)   You exercise regularly, without fail. It's just a habit like any other.

6) Do you keep promises you make to yourself?

    a)   Rarely. Promises are made to be broken!

    b)   Sometimes, especially if you tell other people about them.

    c)   Always. You'd rather die than break your word.

7) There's just enough of your favourite dessert left for one person, and you've already had your share. The rest is being saved for your friend, but your friend has left the room for a few minutes. You:

    a)   Scoff the lot (your friend will never know!).

    b)   Eat half and pretend that's all that was left. Sharing is caring!

    c)   Save it for your friend. There will always be another dessert.

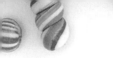

Count up the number of each a) b) and c) answers here:

a)_____

b)_____

c)_____

If you answered all c), you're doing pretty well in the Willpower stakes – nice work! But you wouldn't have picked up this book if you were totally happy with your relationship with sugar, right? So I know you'll be excited to learn you don't have to pile even more responsibility on your Willpower to change that.

If you answered mostly b), you know your Willpower is unreliable at best and you will often try and justify your actions instead of taking responsibility for them. Willpower is a fair-weather friend for you – just like the flaky mate who always bails out on plans at the last minute. The great news is, you don't have to rely on that so-called friend to Outsmart Sugar!

I guess you've already worked out that if you have mostly a) answers, your Willpower could use quite a lot of help! But Willpower doesn't work when it comes to sugar, and here's why:

In my experience, people generally think of Willpower as a finite resource and you only have so much each day to use in your daily battle against the world, including resisting sugary treats. Now I don't know about you, but most people I've come across are using all their Willpower to avoid strangling their boss, their spouse or the guy who cut them off in traffic! So if you have a particularly stressful life and your Willpower is gradually depleted throughout the day by children, managers, significant others, or fellow commuters, your resistance to sugary offerings becomes weaker and weaker.

If you believe in this view of the world, a typical day for a Willpower Warrior might look like this:

…Willpower Warrior starts the day off feeling like a super-hero, full of steely resolve. She laughs in the face of the sugar-bowl, seductively whispering 'just one teaspoon' for her morning coffee. Bypassing the high-sugar cereal and juice, she opts for a satisfying high-protein omelette with that espresso coffee.

Look out! It's the self-appointed office social secretary with chocolate biscuits for morning tea.

Watch it! The charity chocolate box is doing the rounds.

Be vigilant! Stay on the lookout for rogue jars of lollies on desks and countertops.

Pow! Another office birthday cake jumps up.

Lunchtime rolls around and our hero has realised she's made a rookie mistake in not pre-preparing her lunch. Grabbing her bag and carefully considering all the options available to her close-by, she chooses a "healthy" sandwich bar. Here she's offered the add on of a cookie and soft drink for only $2 more by the friendly cashier. Still reeling from

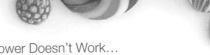

the onslaught of sugar enemies throughout the morning, she says "No, thank you" very politely through gritted teeth. Feeling very impressed with herself, she checks out her Willpower muscles in the shop window and blows them a little kiss in admiration.

Yes! She made it through lunchtime unscathed! But then the dreaded "3pm slump" comes around and our intrepid trooper is fighting hard against it. She digs deep, but her Willpower is weakening against the siren call of a chocolate bar "energy boost". The vending machine calls her name, there's leftover birthday cake in the fridge and those charity chocolates aren't going to buy themselves! In a spirited comeback, she hunts down an apple with almond butter and brews herself an invigorating cup of green tea.

After weaving her way through peak-hour traffic and resisting the urge to stop off at the ice-creamery on the way home, it's dinner time. She collapses on the couch after putting the kids to bed, feeling like she's gone ten rounds with Muhammad Ali. All the fight's gone out of her. Just one square of chocolate won't hurt – she's so worn out she can't resist and, after all, she's been sooooooo good all day! Willpower has deserted her and before she knows it, the whole family block has simply vanished...

And so endeth the sad tale of our Willpower Warrior, defeated and depleted at the end of the day. Some of us don't even make it past morning tea, despite starting out with the very best of intentions. With all the temptations and advertising messages being hurled at us daily, relying on Willpower is foolhardy. It's particularly prone to deserting you when you need it the most – when you're tired or under stress. On top of the usual stress of everyday life, there's a source of fatigue that you probably don't even know about – Decision Fatigue.

Take a guess at how many decisions we make about food in a single day? Five? Ten? Fifteen? My first guess was around twelve, which makes sense when you're just thinking about:

- What shall I eat and drink for breakfast?

- What shall I eat and drink for morning tea?

- What shall I eat and drink for lunch?

- What shall I eat and drink for afternoon tea?

- What shall I eat and drink for dinner?

- What shall I eat and drink after dinner?

Believe it or not, a research project conducted by Professor Brian Wansink of Cornell University, uncovered that we make around two hundred and twenty one decisions *just about food* every single day. That's right – 221, that's not a misprint! We may not be consciously aware of making these food decisions (as you'll soon see, that's where most of the problem lies!) but, combined with the hundreds of other decisions you need to make each day, this leads to Decision Fatigue.

Think about every single decision or choice you have to make in a day, whether it be conscious or not…

- Can I hit the snooze button one more time?

- Should I go to the gym or sleep in another 45 minutes?

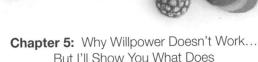

Chapter 5: Why Willpower Doesn't Work...
But I'll Show You What Does

- Will I do weights or cardio when I go to the gym?

- Should I check my phone/emails before or after getting into the shower?

- What perfume/aftershave will I wear today?

- What colour socks will I wear today?

- Which shoes will I wear today?

- What dress/suit/jeans/shirt will I wear today?

- What will I pack for the kids' lunches today?

- Do I have any leftovers from dinner I can take for lunch today?

- What will I have for breakfast today?

- Will I have tea or coffee with my breakfast today?

- Do I actually have time for breakfast?

- If not, do I have enough cash to grab a coffee and muffin from the cafe next to work that doesn't take credit cards?

- Should I fill the car up with petrol on the way to or from work?

Feeling overwhelmed yet? And we still haven't even gotten out of bed! Every single one of these questions demands your attention and energy, whether you're aware of it or not.

Most of us think about decisions in light of BIG, potentially life-changing choices…

• What university to apply for…

• What job to take…

• What suburb to live in…

• Whether to buy a house or an apartment…

• Who to marry…

• When to have children and how many…

…and so on. The really big decisions only have to be made once or twice in your life (unless you're Elizabeth Taylor!) but the daily grind of choosing between many options wears us out. This is what truly depletes our Willpower, and by much more than we realise.

Now, because Willpower is simply the ability to resist short-term temptation for long-term gain, the way your brain works sets you up for failure before you even begin! How exactly? Well, "Now You" thinks of "Future You" as a totally different person. Brain scans show that totally separate parts light up when we're asked to think of ourselves and when we're asked to think of someone else. This is logical, because this means you're pre-programmed to take care of yourself first. The interesting part is that when you're asked to think of "Future You", most people's brain lights up in the part for *other* people. No wonder it's so hard for "Now You" to use Willpower to resist temptation now for "Future You". You have no loyalty whatsoever to his strange person, even though logically

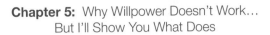

you know you should be looking out for them. Subconsciously, your brain has no sympathy for anyone other than yourself and just wants to enjoy that doughnut that "Now You" really wants!

Willpower relies on resisting what you DON'T want

Besides being depleted by the decision fatigue, another reason Willpower doesn't work is that it that it focuses our brain on what we DON'T want in order to create a plan to avoid it. We have to think about it first and, in the words of so many philosophers and self-help gurus, "What we focus on expands". Let's try a simple little exercise to demonstrate just how counter-productive this is…

… I want you to create a picture in your mind of a pink fluffy toy bunny. The pinker and fluffier the better – imagine his cute button nose, his adorable cotton tail and big doe eyes. Imagine cuddling him to your chest and feeling the fuzzy fur tickle your nose. Close your eyes for a moment and really let that image take hold in your mind. A totally clear image of the most loveable, huggable pink fluffy toy bunny.

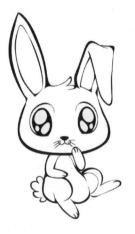

OK, now stop thinking about the pink fluffy bunny. Think about any other thing you like – anything at all, but just DON'T think of the pink fluffy bunny. Use all of your powers of concentration to eliminate all traces of the pink fluffy bunny from your mind. You shouldn't be seeing the pink fluffy bunny at all now and you certainly shouldn't be thinking about how nice it felt to hug that adorable little pink fluffy bunny. Resist thinking of the pink fluffy bunny NOW!!

Did it work? Could you stop thinking of the pink fluffy bunny when I asked you to resist thinking about him? Of course not, because it's impossible – our brains just don't work that way. Unfortunately, the same happens when we try to force ourselves NOT to think of the rest of the family block of chocolate in the pantry, or the tub of caramel swirl ice-cream sitting unfinished in the freezer. Attempting to suppress thoughts actually makes them stronger.

Trying to banish certain things from our consciousness is a futile exercise, because our brain simply doesn't have a mechanism for doing it. It's just another way our brain messes with us – after all, the only way to know for sure that you're NOT thinking about a pink fluffy bunny is by monitoring thoughts and scanning for any traces of said bunny. So the process basically goes like this:

"Am I thinking about an adorable pink fluffy bunny?"

"Well, I wasn't, but now I am …"

Psychologists call this an ironic thought process. This explains why you only want the stuff that you "can't" have, why trying to suppress laughter only makes you laugh more and why you fall flat on your face when you're trying to impress someone (or reverse your car into a mailbox… ask me about that one when we meet!) and so on. It also helps to explain why some people find it easy to avoid sugar…

…because they're not actually thinking about it!

I'll let that one sink in just a little bit.

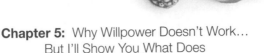

Chapter 5: Why Willpower Doesn't Work…
But I'll Show You What Does

So, what can we do about your depleting Willpower? Stop worrying about it for a start! Another weapon is copying what highly successful people do. Don't worry, copying stopped being a sin once you left school! If you want great results, find someone who does what you want to do and just do that – this is called "modelling".

Regardless of what you think of his political views, I suspect Barack Obama probably had quite a bit more on his "to-do" list as President of the USA than the average human – don't you? So how do you free up enough brain power to focus on being the most powerful man running the most influential country in the world? It all comes down to limiting choice wherever and whenever possible. Mr Obama has been quoted as saying "I don't want to make decisions about what I'm eating or wearing, because I have too many other decisions to make".

Take notice next time you see footage of President Obama - does that outfit look just a little familiar? Choosing to wear the same style of tie and blue or grey suit every day frees your mind from having to make a whole lot of micro-decisions every day. Scheduling exercise at same time every day and eating the same breakfast at the same time every day? This is exactly what Barack Obama does to ensure he sets himself up for success every day. Wow – there goes at least another fifty micro-decisions!

Can you see how modelling the President of the USA might help you to Outsmart Sugar? By building in your own safeguards and reducing the number of micro-decisions you make every day, you leave less to chance and momentary weakness. But how exactly do we do this without a team of advisors? Before you've finished this book, I'll show you exactly the methods I use so you can create your very own Personal Policies, tactics and strategies.

CHAPTER 6

NEVER SAY DIE(T)!

"Diets are boring and so are people talking about them."

— Mireille Guiliano

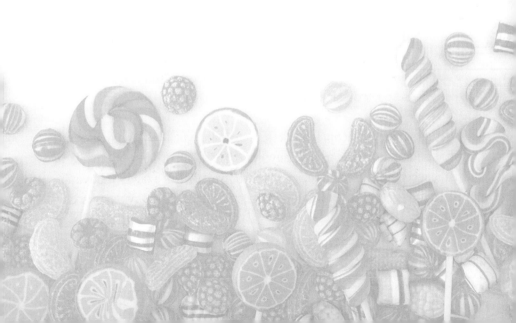

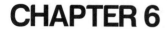

CHAPTER 6

NEVER SAY DIE(T)!

"Ice-cream is short-sighted escapism."
— Tara Mitchell

In the famous words of one of my favourite cartoon characters, Garfield, and emblazoned on fridge magnets the world over "Diet is DIE with a T". If the thought of a diet sends you running for the hills – GOOD! A diet conjures up all sorts of negative images – highly restricted, often quite weird food combinations, all designed to get you to lose weight FAST. If you're a normal human being (and I assume you are!) the restrictive nature of these diets will have your inner rebel screaming out for what you "can't" have. And you know from the last chapter how well that goes!

Restrictions only serve to form enemies between your mind and body. Dieting, restricting or giving up certain foods implies lack and humans are conditioned to gorge when we perceive lack. Our prehistoric "Lizard Brain" will order the body to stuff itself silly and hang on to body fat for dear life when it appears that there may be an upcoming famine. This is true even in today's world where an abundance of food is only a phone call, mouse-click or car-trip away.

The reason most people don't lose weight when following diets is because nobody likes to lose anything. Think about those moments of panic when you lose your keys, phone or wallet? Not exactly motivating is it? It might even conjure up images of your Grade Five sports day,

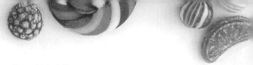

when you ran your little heart out in the 100 metre sprint, but lost to that damn Pat Jones that always beat you at everything else, plus was better-looking and had better hair and... oh, sorry, maybe that was just me!

Losing at anything knocks your self-esteem, especially when you have so much of your self-image tied up in it – as the dieting industry spends millions on making you believe. The in-built failure mechanism with almost all diets is the focus on losing weight, rather than achieving a lifestyle outcome. They also direct your complete attention onto what you *can't* have – you will inevitably fail because it requires you to do the one thing that guarantees failure - that is, thinking about all of the sugary stuff you're trying to avoid! You know from the previous chapter on Willpower that trying not to think about something will actually intensify your thoughts of whatever it is you're trying not to think about.

You also know from Chapter 2 that when the bigger and more dramatic the effect, the more you sit up and take notice. That's why these fad or celebrity-endorsed diets sell so well – the advertising is extremely high impact and very easy to manipulate. Take any celebrity who's slimmed down for a movie role – all you see is the before and after pictures. You don't see the weeks and often months of nutritionally-perfect food intake, hard work and exercise that it really takes for long-term change. They can stick to it because they have a very specific outcome coupled with a very specific date by which to achieve that outcome. If you had to get naked for a movie role, I bet you could stick to any crazy "diet" in the world! But it would only be short term fix, not a long term healthy lifestyle.

What will really make the difference in your life is deciding to Outsmart Sugar as a way of life, not part of a "diet". The below diet has been doing the rounds on the internet for years now. Whilst it's quite humorous, it's a classic demonstration of how stress increases through the day when you deprive yourself:

"Daily Stress" Diet
A diet designed to help with the stress that builds up during the day.

BREAKFAST
1/2 grapefruit
1 slice wholemeal toast (no butter)
1 cup of skimmed milk

LUNCH
1 small, lean boiled chicken breast
1 large serve of steamed spinach
1 glass of unsweetened fruit juice
1 chocolate digestive biscuit

MID-AFTERNOON SNACK
Rest of biscuits in packet
Family sized tub of chocolate chip ice-cream with hot fudge sauce

DINNER
2 loaves garlic bread with cheese
Large pizza with the lot
Large chips
Family sized block of milk chocolate
1/2 bottle wine

LATE EVENING SNACK
Rest of bottle of wine
Entire frozen Black Forest Gateau

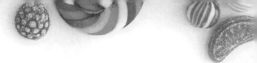

Chapter 6: Never Say Die(t)!

I know you're probably having a giggle to yourself right now and thinking "Well, that escalated quickly!" Although this amusing snapshot of a single day in a dieter's life may not be typical, if you stretch the time period out a bit longer, it's almost exactly what happens longer term. How many people do you know who've slimmed down for a specific event (weddings are the quintessential illustration of this – there's an entire industry set up around helping brides get "wedding-weight" ready!) or reached a goal weight, then go straight back to their old habits and pile all the weight back on again?

You're set up for failure with these diets and they're specifically designed to keep you on the weight-loss roundabout. Either you fail spectacularly (like the above tongue in cheek example) which causes you to feel bad about yourself, lower your self-esteem and set you back on the spiral downwards and searching for yet another quick fix. Or, you do really well for a short period of time, achieve your goal, then go back to your old habits and pile the weight back on. Once again, you feel like a failure. Diets are, by their very nature and design, unsustainable. They push you into behaviour that's not usual or normal for you and you want to go running back to your comfort zone as soon as possible. They're a temporary measure and never meant for any commitment longer than a few weeks at most.

The euphemistically named "Weight Management" industry (in other words, sales of services and products that are designed to either help you get skinny or ripped!) was recently valued at over $590 Billion US Dollars. Yes, that's right - Billion with a "B". This kind of revenue isn't generated by people trying things once, getting the result they want, and going on their merry way. All of these companies want you as a repeat customer and they have the marketing budget to buy the celebrity endorsements and advertising to get it.

No-one goes to sleep and wakes up obese, but our modern quick-fix world, we are conditioned to believe the company or celebrity that tells us we can lose the weight gained over months or even years in 7, 14 or 30 days.

"Drop A Dress Size in Just One Week!!" scream the tabloids!!

"Bust Your Gut – Quick-Hit Strategies to Kill the Beer Belly" shouts the latest men's fitness and health magazine!!

Of course, word-of-mouth is the most powerful form of endorsement and no-one is better (or more aggressive!) at this than MLM's (Multi-Level Marketing) companies.

I was asked by a friend of mine to join one of these network marketing companies, which sells itself as being at the forefront of health, and offers amazing opportunities for those who sign up to create a significant residual income for themselves. You of course, have to sell bucket loads of bars, shakes and other strange meal-replacements subscriptions so you can keep that cash rolling in. They use the classic "Before" and "After" shots that illustrate to you in an instant just how ripped you can get in four weeks. What is written in very, very small print, is the expectation that you will work out like a maniac and your intake of real food is highly restricted and regulated. You don't see or experience the hard work that goes on in-between the two photos and of course there are some very clever lighting and contouring tricks that can be employed in the absence of Photoshop to enhance both shots.

Being the curious individual that I am, my very first port of call was to check the ingredient lists of the products I'd be heartily endorsing to my friends and family. I was shocked (but not entirely surprised) that sugar

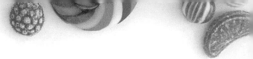

in her various disguises, was in the top four ingredients of just about every single product in the very, very vast range of Frankenfoods. It seems that the high level of sugar is just there to replace the energy that you'd normally get from eating real food – and to fuel all those insane gym workouts!

Frightening stuff, but if you're as smart as I know you are, you'll see right through this type of marketing and always, always check the label. Next time you're in the Supermarket, take a quick look at the ingredients list on any type of "diet" or indeed "muscle" or "protein" shake. I'm willing to bet my house that sugar or one of its aliases will be in the top four ingredients, right at the top of a scarily long list of other, often unpronounceable ingredients. This is the simplest way to Outsmart those diet companies who're spending millions of dollars trying to convince you they're here to "help" you. Just one look at the ingredients list panel will persuade you otherwise.

Think you're immune to such blatant false advertising? It can be far more insidious than that. Perhaps you might read with interest about a celebrity following a macrobiotic diet, which makes her look and feel amazing (just check out the Photoshopped images on the front of the glossy magazine for proof!) Or another who sings the praises of the Lemon Detox Diet, that helped them lose weight for their latest film role. You saw that film and yes, they did appear to have lost a lot of weight in the semi-naked love scenes. We seem to forget the article we read about the body-double who works out eight hours a day to make their living as the on-camera naked backside of Mr or Mrs Hollywood!

Rich and famous, being paid millions to star in movies or endorse products and gadding about via first-class air travel, snapping up the best tables at the hottest restaurants, the most fabulous holidays in exotic locations and strutting the red carpet in the latest designer outfits. Who wouldn't want that? The implication is that these celebrities are the Alpha Males and Females of humanity - they live the life that we all aspire to. Although you might not have their acting or singing talent (or no discernible talent at all, in the case of certain celebrities!) you can still get a piece of their action by following their diet.

However close you think you might be getting to being a real-life movie-star by following their diet, you will inevitably desert it after a while. Attempting to follow these regimes without the assistance of a full-time team of a personal chef, house cleaner, trainer, life-coach, nanny, talent agent, security guard and driver is a recipe for failure – and that's exactly how they're designed. To make you feel even worse, celebrities claim they're just like everyone else, doing their best to appear likeable, accessible and "human" (which of course, is just a tactic to ensure their ongoing popularity and keep on selling movies/concerts/TV shows/ music). So in "failing" in something so basic as following the way another fellow human being eats, any belief that you could possibly be in the same league as them is shaken. Your self-esteem takes a massive blow. So you go looking for the next quick-fix, which will give you a fleeting sense of being back in control.

Now this is where I find it gets really interesting. Even though the celebrity lifestyle we aspire to looks amazing from the outside, we know that it can be devastating for some – you just need to look at the string of suicides, "accidental" car crashes, publicly humiliating mental breakdowns and outbreaks, as well as multiple divorces, "kiss-and-tell" exposés and stories of paparazzi harassment to see the fall-out from fame and fortune. There's also the legendary casting couch, from where we hear tales of young starlets doing just about anything just to get cast in a TV show or movie. Subconsciously, we don't actually want any of this. Why would anyone want a life where stalking and insane invasions of privacy aren't criminal acts, but acceptable practices?

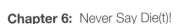

Even if they haven't been involved in any scandals or released a sex-tape, we know that celebrities' amazing bodies probably aren't thanks to drinking nothing but lemon juice, cayenne pepper and maple syrup for a month. They're more than likely following a highly-disciplined work-out routine and carefully monitoring their food intake. Our conscious desire to be "just like them" is tempered by the fact we really do know the truth deep down.

At the core, I believe this is the real reason celebrity diets fail – not only are they unsustainable, but they are at odds with our subconscious beliefs. This disconnect between subconscious and conscious is where the source of discomfort comes from. Eventually, we settle back to our comfort zone, because our subconscious is actually a little bit frightened of what we might really have to do to be "just like" that celebrity!

Rather than blindly following the latest celebrity diet promoted by whoever's "Banging Beach Body" is gracing the cover of the glossies this week and continuing on that self-esteem roller-coaster, wouldn't you rather be able to dismiss sugary crap easily and effortlessly and feel great about being You?

The Triple E - Easy Esteem Exercise

Feeling a bit flat after seeing too many "Perfect (read: Airbrushed!) Beach Bodies" on the cover of magazines? Then let me show you a way to boost your self-esteem so you feel much better about yourself and start acting like it too!

Firstly, stop for a moment and vividly imagine your natural, confident self. That's the one! You already know how easy it is to be confident – you've done it all your life.

Now, step into that supremely confident posture. Remember what your mum told you –

– Shoulders back!

– Spine straight!

– Chest out!

– Chin up!

Now, tell me - what do you say to yourself when you're confident? What's your War Cry? It might just be a simple "YES!!" or "(Insert your favourite profanity here) YEAH!" Write it down here, so you can come back to it if you need to:

Now, clench your fist and thrust it either straight up in the air or out in front of you, the choice is yours.

Now, do it again, this time yelling your War Cry.

Again – this time like you mean it!!

One more time – even louder and more courageous than before!

How does that feel?

Better?

I thought so.

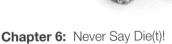

The Short-circuit EEE

Haven't got time for the full-size EEE or maybe you're in the middle of a crowded Supermarket?

How about an instant burst of confidence in less than three seconds? Your wish is my command!

Remember how we talked about how Sugar messes with your Bio-feedback in Chapter 3? This is how you can turn the tables and use Bio-feedback to your advantage. When you physically STAND like you're confident, you automatically FEEL like you're confident. Here's how:

- Stand up.

- Place your fingertips on your sternum (right in the centre of your chest).

- Take a deep breath in - make your hand move up and out by at least five centimetres.

Notice how your posture straightens up, you're standing straighter and feeling taller.

Bam!

Instant confidence and self-esteem right there!

You're welcome.

CHAPTER 7

DIRTY MARKETING TRICKS AND HOW TO OUTSMART THEM

"A market is never saturated
with a good product,
but it is very quickly
saturated with a bad one."

— Henry Ford

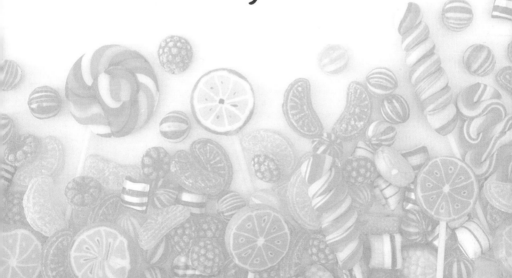

CHAPTER 7

DIRTY MARKETING TRICKS AND HOW TO OUTSMART THEM

"Food Manufacturers don't care about your health, they only care whether you're a repeat customer."
— Tara Mitchell

You already know all about the sugar in muesli bars, chocolate bars, breakfast cereals, jam and "low-fat" yoghurt. But next time you go to the Supermarket (or even open your pantry door!) check the ingredients list on savoury foods like:

- Tomato Sauce
- Tomato Paste
- Barbecue Sauce
- Curry Paste
- Salad Dressings
- Bread
- Baked Beans
- Mayonnaise
- Canned Vegetables

- Pickled Vegetables
- Canned fish
- Chutney
- Marinades
- Glazes
- Flavoured Vinegar
- Spice Mixes
- Crushed Garlic

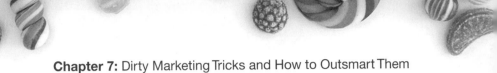

Many of these have sugar listed in the top three ingredients – even supposedly one-ingredient products like crushed garlic! Food Manufacturers know that sugar can make almost anything more attractive to the human palate, so you're more likely to buy it again.

And again.

And again.

Despite what they tell you in their advertising, Food Manufacturers definitely do not have your best interests at heart.

They don't care about your health.

They don't care about your kids' health.

They don't care whether you have more time to spend with your family.

Their sole mission: create brand loyalty and get you to repeatedly buy their product instead of their competitors. That's it!

Food Manufacturers and Supermarkets work hard to program your brain, imprinting their brands on your consciousness and manipulating your beliefs. Here are just some of the tactics they use and ways you can Outsmart them.

Celebrity Endorsement

Ever since there's been stage, screen and music celebrities, there's been celebrity endorsement. Why? Because it works! Humans instinctively distrust anything that's different to what we're used to, because in our lunch-hunting days that could mean something (or someone!) dangerous had intruded on our tribe. A celebrity helps make the unfamiliar familiar and "safe" to us, lowering our defences. You might never have seen the product before, but you know and like the face promoting it. Attaching familiarity to a product reduces any anxiety or stress we might feel about buying that product. Celebrity Chefs have a whole new career path that didn't exist ten years ago – they're now endorsing products and Supermarkets like it's going out of fashion!

Advertisers also know we're buying a tiny bit of celebrity lifestyle when we buy the products they endorse. I may not have George Clooney's mansion by Lake Como, but I can drink the same pod coffee he does (***Disclaimer: George Clooney may or may not actually drink pod coffee).

When you see these ads, whether on a screen or in print, remember that they're really just highly-produced, miniature pieces of art. Thinking of them this way and appreciating them for their entertainment value alone will help reduce their influence on you.

The Guilt Factor

As if we don't have enough to be guilty about (that reminds me, I must call Mum & Dad...) boxed chocolate manufacturers have harnessed guilt as their weapon of choice. Their entire marketing strategy is based around two basic themes:

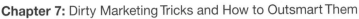

A) You are a bad guest if you show up to someone's house for a Lunch/ Dinner/BBQ without a box of chocolates

B) You are a bad person if you do not say Sorry/Happy Birthday/Happy Anniversary/Valentine's Day with a box of chocolates

Like me, if you were brought up proper and wouldn't dream of turning up to someone's house empty-handed, you're probably thinking "But what would I take instead of chocolate?"

Here's a few ideas....

- Upmarket Mineral Water

- Flowers

- House plant

- Loaf of Specialty Bread

- Fruit Platter

- Dips

- Spiced Nuts

- Homemade Preserves or Sauce

- Cheese

- Local Olive Oil and Flavoured Vinegar

- Craft Beer

- Small-batch Spirits

- Wine

See, there are plenty of other things you can bring – most of which you can also pick up at the last minute and are far more interesting than that boring box of chocolates!

Emotional Product Placement

Some product placements are pretty obvious, like the brands of cars used in movie car-chases or high-sugar cereal advertised during kids' TV shows. What's less obvious is mood-based product placement. What does this mean for you? Well, think about how you feel when you watch a typical news broadcast, telling you about war, murders, kidnappings and the latest stock market crash. If you're anything like me, you might feel a little…

… sad

… hopeless

… useless

… powerless

… cynical about humanity

…all of which lead to you being pretty despondent about the future, don't you agree? This makes you care even less than you already do about "Future You" - and you already know how this affects your Willpower! Fast Food manufactures love to advertise to you when you're in this frame of mind. When your future looks so hopeless, it doesn't really matter if you stuff your face with ALL the bad foods right now, because we could all die tomorrow!

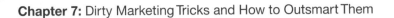

The best way to Outsmart this kind of advertising is simply to be mindful of your emotions and moods. I'll give you some great tips on how to do this in Chapter 10, Manage Your Mind - Mindfully!

The 3pm "Slump"

We all know (because we've been told to!) we should be feeling low and listless in the mid-afternoon. Although there's some evidence your body naturally has a mid-afternoon energy dip, it's far more likely you've set yourself up with a sugar high-crash-high cycle. And don't the chocolate and biscuit manufacturers just love capitalising on this – it's a self-perpetuating cycle, a marketers dream!

Sugar is being employed here as a form of mind control. It keeps you at your desk when it's scientifically proven taking a walk or doing a few jumping jacks will give you healthier and longer-lasting energy.

You can Outsmart this one very easily by eating well throughout the day and always having a decent breakfast. Check out the website **outsmartsugarnow.com** for more suggestions or simply make a commitment to having a Green Smoothie every day. My Simple Starter Formula for the perfect Green Smoothie is in the very last Chapter for you.

Manufactured Sugar-Giving Occasions

Did you know American candy producers actually attempted to launch "National Candy Day" in 1916? This was before they hit on the goldmine that is Trick or Treating in the USA. This holiday dwarfs all others for manufactured sugar sales – almost 300 million kilos of the stuff is sold in the last week of October. That's almost one kilo for every man, woman and child! Thankfully, we're not quite at that point in Australia (yet), but you can bet it won't be far off.

St Valentine's Day was declared in the year 496, but it didn't have any romantic connotations until the late Middle Ages. The first heart-shaped Valentine's Day box of chocolates was introduced by Cadbury (who else?!) in 1868. Since then, it's been compulsory to give your sweetheart chocolates, and 35 million boxes of them are sold around the world on Valentine's Day every year.

Eggs have been a symbol of new life for millennia, but it wasn't until our old friends Cadbury came up with hollow chocolate eggs in 1875 that sugar became entwined with them. By 1893, they had 19 different patents for Easter chocolate designs – which gives you some idea of how valuable the connection is! In Britain, the Cadbury Creme Egg is the single-biggest confectionary seller between New Year's Day and Easter. Interestingly, Cadbury have decreed it may only be on the shelves for this period. Why do they need up to four months to sell a product that's supposed to be eaten on one day only?? It's not really about Easter now, is it?

Celebrations of all kinds have been overrun with sugar commercialism, which has clouded their origins and history. Even if you're not religious, I'm sure you'll agree there's more to Christmas and Easter than chocolate Advent Calendars and eggs! Outsmart the Food Manufacturers by making these kinds of events special again in your own way – create your own family traditions or borrow some from other cultures.

"Sales"

Even though online shopping means we have an entire world of products at our fingertips 24/7, the mere mention of the word "sale" can still whip people into a frenzy! Why? Remember back in our lunch-chasing days, it was feast or famine. "Sales" tap into our primordial belief that if

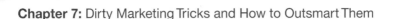

something is scarce, we damn well better make sure and grab as much of it as possible before it disappears and we're starving again. This is known as "Scarcity Mentality" but the crowd who love an acronym know it as "FOMO": Fear Of Missing Out.

Of course, you're far too smart to join those silly people lining up at 1am on Boxing Day just to get a good deal on a toaster. But Food Manufacturers and Supermarkets are very good at invoking the scarcity mentality in you without you even being aware of it... until you've loaded up your trolley with ten family-sized blocks of chocolate!

To Outsmart the artificial time-pressure from "sales", do this: Every time you feel like scooping up armfuls of sugary sale items, remind yourself of this mantra:

There's plenty more – there will always be another one out there.

Lighting

Supermarket shopping is stressful! Before you've even set foot in the store, you've had to compete for a car park and physically wrestle with a trolley that wants to go in any direction but straight ahead. At last, you reach the bright, welcoming lights of the store – illuminating all those wonderful products to maximise your convenience! That's the message the Supermarkets want you to receive, but bright lights are actually a highly effective tool in controlling you once you enter the Supermarket.

Your brain relies on feedback from your body to tell it what to think. It's scientifically proven that when you smile, your brain thinks you're happy – because you only smile when you're happy, right? This is another example of Bio-feedback. When there's a bright light, you squint. Squinting looks a lot like the face you pull when you're worried or stressed. So guess how your brain interprets that bit of Bio-feedback? Yep – it believes you're stressed. Just to add to the tension you had before you even walked in the store! This is where all the Food Manufacturers' advertising really pays off - you'll head straight to the sugary foods that help you to "relax", "escape" or "take a break".

If you really want to Outsmart this bit of Bio-feedback, wear sunglasses when you shop!

Priming

Let me ask you something: How often do you buy flowers from the Supermarket?

a)   Regularly – it's part of my weekly shop.

b)   Sometimes – if I've forgotten a birthday!

c)   Rarely or never

If you're like most people, the answer is c). Yet every major Supermarket has fresh flowers at the entrance to the store, along with huge displays of fruit, vegetables and loaves of bread. Because these are all highly perishable, your brain "knows" they must be fresh and therefore everything else in the store must also be fresh. This is called "priming" and it relies on the fact that first impressions count to the human brain.

Another way you can be "primed" is through your sense of smell. Have you noticed that almost all Supermarkets have bakeries and hot roast

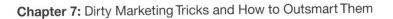

chickens now? Those delicious smells mean you'll start salivating and guess what? Your brain takes that as Biofeedback and thinks you're hungry, even if you've just eaten. You're also far more open to suggestion, so those huge displays of stuff on "sale" look like more of a bargain.

I'm going to bet you already know how to Outsmart this one – never go shopping on an empty stomach!

Your Own Imagination

As we've talked about before – your brain is sometimes your own worst enemy. Food Manufacturers and Supermarkets know exactly how to harness your imagination and use it against you. Just seeing products on the shelf can set your mind racing, thinking about the luxurious creaminess of ice-cream or the silky milk chocolate dissolving in your mouth.

Droooooool...

...oops, sorry!!

A great way to Outsmart this one is to chew gum whilst you shop. This distracts your brain and makes it almost impossible to imagine another food in your mouth. But please, learn to chew it elegantly, with your mouth closed and not imitating a cow chewing cud!

Labels

The "Low-fat" cult is one of the biggest scams pulled off in human food history. Low-fat inevitably means high-sugar. Don't fall for it. Fat means flavour (ask any chef!) and there is more and more evidence that sugar is the devil for your health, not fat. By removing fat, flavour is also removed and something else needs to be added to make it more palatable. And guess what's Number One in attractiveness to the human palate?

Sugar!

Now, of course Food Manufacturers know that high levels of sweetness appeal to us. They also know it's not cool to have the word 'sugar' listed on the label, so they'll go to great lengths to disguise it. One easy way to find sugar on a label is to keep an eye out for anything ending in '–ose', like:

- Sucrose

- Maltose

- Dextrose

- Fructose

- Glucose

- Galactose

- Lactose

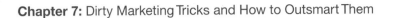

But there are also many other types of sugar, some of which even sound healthy, like:

- Agave Nectar

- Organic Brown Sugar

- Corn Syrup

- Dehydrated Fruit Juice

Some Food Manufacturers even use several different types of sugar together, so each individual one is listed much further down the list of ingredients. At first glance, it might look like you're eating a low-sugar product – don't fall for it!

To completely Outsmart the Food Manufacturers, buy fresh produce that doesn't even have labels! But when you do buy packaged food, watch out for the "–ose's" and the huge number of other names sugar goes by – I've listed them for your convenience on the website **outsmartsugarnow.com.**

Also, be sure and check out the Nutrition Information Panel on the label – it will tell you how many grams of sugar are there. Most packaged food contains more than one single serve (sorry, one family block of chocolate does NOT equal one serve!!) so take care and read the column that says 'per serve' not 'per 100g' or 'per pack'.

Remember that 4 grams = 1 teaspoon of sugar and it's recommended that we keep it to 6 to 9 teaspoons per day, or 24 to 36 grams. Now might be a good time to flip back to the start of Chapter 3, where you wrote down your daily sugar intake and see where you're at.

Checkout Design

Have you ever been waiting on a checkout line, looked down at your basket and thought "Yeah, I don't really need that family-sized bag of "fun-sized" bars"? Good luck trying to find somewhere to put it down – checkouts are designed so you can't. Most people won't turn around and put it back, they'll just buy it. We don't like to be wrong and with all those people and cameras around, your 'wrong' choice is obvious to everyone.

Smart-tip: No-one is watching you, unless you're trying to stuff that bag under your jumper! If you find something in your basket or trolley that doesn't belong there: PUT IT BACK!

And then there are the "impulse" displays – glossy magazines, chocolate bars plus all manner of chewing gum, mints and tiny gadgets stacked ever so temptingly at eye-level at the checkout. Even at the self-serve checkouts, there are waist-high baskets filled to bursting with sugary confection on "sale". Obviously, Supermarkets know you'll see them whilst you're queuing up – even if you're staring at your phone the whole time, your peripheral vision will pick them up. Admit it: you've absentmindedly grabbed something from the checkout line at some point. I know I have. It won't come as a surprise to you that a whopping 80% of sugary confection purchases are unplanned!

Being Mindful when shopping is a great way to Outsmart this. Always be completely present when you're shopping, not focussed on something else. I'll share some great tips on how to do this shortly.

If you can, shop without the kids – that's who the Supermarkets are really targeting with impulse displays. I know this isn't always possible,

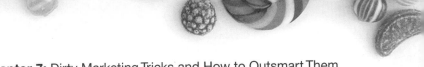

so my tip to help kids Outsmart Supermarkets is to write a shopping list together. Then get your kids to help fetch things and tick them off the list. Turning the shopping into a treasure hunt makes it fun and, with a bit of luck, they'll be so focussed on the adventure, they won't even see the impulse display!

The Shortcut

Want to know the single easiest way to Outsmart Food Manufacturers?

JERF

No, I'm not calling you names or telling you where to go, I promise! JERF stands for:

JUST
EAT
REAL
FOOD

Pretty simple really. If you choose real, unprocessed food over sugar and additive-laden, packaged crap, you can Outsmart ALL the hidden sugars - and you don't even have to think about it!

How's that for reducing your Decision Fatigue?

CHAPTER 8

PERSONAL POLICY MAKING 101

"Make your own rules or be a slave to another's."

— William Blake

CHAPTER 8

PERSONAL POLICY MAKING 101

"It's Your life – You decide The Rules. Game on!"
– Tara Mitchell

The phrase "Policy Making" might conjure up visions of politicians in blue suits deciding on what's best for the nation without your input or involvement. However, everyone has their own Personal Policies that they live by. For example, do any of these sound familiar to you?

1. If I eat a chocolate bar and no-one saw me eat it, it never happened.

2. Always have a Diet Coke with a Mars Bar, as the calories of the Mars Bar are cancelled out by the Diet Coke.

3. Sugar for medicinal purposes doesn't count e.g. barley sugar sweets and hot chocolate.

4. Foods that from part of an entertainment package, such as ice-cream at the cinema or chocolate eaten while watching TV or videos with other people, are part of the shared experience and therefore do not count.

5. Foods of the same colour are considered to be similarly healthy e.g. mushrooms and white chocolate, spinach and pistachio ice-cream.

6. Always break sweet biscuits in half before eating. Breaking them causes all the calories to leak out.

7. Things licked off knives and teaspoons whilst you are in the process of preparing something e.g. cake frosting or cookie dough, do not count.

8. Movies are incomplete without Jaffas (or Fantales, or a giant Coke, or a choc-top ice-cream or....).

9. Dairy is good for you. Ice-cream is dairy. Therefore, ice-cream for breakfast is a great way of getting healthy!

I'm betting you've used at least one of these to justify your consumption of sugar! Don't feel bad about it – trust me, I've used all of these and made up at least ten more on the fly in order to make myself feel better.

Whilst the above was quite light-hearted, there are also Personal Policies that can quite literally save your life, such as:

1. Always do up your seatbelt when travelling in a car.

2. Obey STOP signs at intersections.

3. Avoid walking down dark alley-ways on your own at night.

4. Look both ways before crossing the street.

4. Don't stand under tall trees in a lightning storm.

5. Swim between the flags at the beach.

Outsmarting Sugar may not have the instantaneous impact that, say, avoiding a car accident does. But the long-term effects of sugar can be just as devastating on your health, as we saw in Chapter 3 "What Sugar Really Does to Your Body…". It's just as important to make Personal Policies about what you put into your body as it is to avoid immediately life-threatening situations.

Creating your own set of rules might sound awfully restrictive at first, but please hear me out. Doing this will actually result in you making smarter choices with minimal effort. Think about every sport or game that there is. How would you be able to play or know whether you'd won or lost if you didn't know the rules?

By creating and articulating your Personal Policies precisely and clearly, they become your very own game rules and you'll know when you're winning! The best part is that they will reduce and perhaps even totally eliminate the need to think about Every. Single. Decision. you're faced with when it comes to your sugar intake.

A good place to start is identifying the top five times that you feel you "need" sugar. Write them down here:

1. _____

2. _____

3. _____

4. _____

5. _____

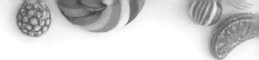

Everyone's list will be different but, in my experience, all responses can be sorted into the five categories below. To help you classify your answers, I've provided some common statements that help illustrate the types of situations:

Energy. I need six teaspoons of sugar in my coffee just to get out the door!

Habit. I *always* have dessert after dinner!

Mindlessness. I sat down in front of the TV with the intention of just having one square of chocolate... wait, where did that whole family-sized block go??!!

Peer Pressure. I feel like I'm not celebrating 'properly' if I don't eat the cake!

Emotional. I'm feeling bored/stressed/upset/heartbroken/sad and I want a distraction.

Now that you know the five main categories where most people believe they "need" sugar, go ahead and classify those five times you wrote down above. This will help you identify where you need the most help in creating your Personal Policies, especially if a category pops up several times for you.

1. _____

Category_____

2. _____

Category_____

3. _____

Category_____

4. _____

Category_____

5. _____

Category_____

www.OutsmartSugarNow.com

OK, cool – we've worked out some trigger points for you now. So how is Personal Policy making going to help you here? Well, you already know that Willpower is simply not enough, especially when you're tired, hungry or time-pressured. Your Personal Policies are going to back you up, so you don't have to rely on Willpower.

You also already know that Food Manufacturers and Supermarkets are doing their best to brainwash you into automatically buying processed junk. Your Personal Policies can help here too, by short-circuiting your automatic responses before they even make you take action.

However, where I believe Personal Policies are going to help you most of all is with the greatest enabler there is. This is the one that is constantly with you, the one that will always say "Yes!" to sugar, the one that it's impossible to escape from. Who is it? Let me introduce you to...

You.

Or, more specifically, your Inner Child.

If you've ever spent any time around small children (or even if you've been one!), you'll know that they don't take "No" for an answer easily. They also have no concept of the future or of the consequences of their actions. You've no doubt also noted they have absolutely no shame and are highly skilled negotiators! You don't stand a chance without some firm rules in place. Your Inner Child is no different.

A simple "I just need to pop in to grab something for dinner" trip to the Supermarket alone is fraught with danger. Not only do you have to contend with all the Dirty Marketing Tricks the Food Manufacturers and Supermarkets are throwing at you, your Inner Child will push you towards rash decisions!

If yours is anything like mine used to be, your internal conversation at the Supermarket might go a little something like this...

You: Righto, just ducking in to pick up something for dinner. Veggie stir-fry I think, or maybe an omelette, perhaps chicken and... something? I'll just see what takes my fancy.

Inner Child: Ooooh, look at the pretty colourful packets in the middle aisles!! Let's go see what's new and exciting!!

You: Maybe I'll just grab one small bar of chocolate, it's been a tough day.

Inner Child: Ooooh, look the BIG block has a red tag on it!!

You: Well, I AM frugal and sensible – the family size is 15c per 100g cheaper, so it really doesn't make economic sense to buy the smaller packet.

Inner Child: I am smart and good at math!!

You: I won't open it 'til I get home and share with husband/wife/kids/housemate.

Inner Child: Open it! Open it! Open it!

You: Well, I am a little tired after a long day. Maybe just one piece - I deserve it!

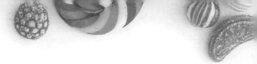

Inner Child: I am a good girl/boy and I deserve a treat!!

Most of the packet is mindlessly eaten whilst you reflect on your current Personal Policy that it doesn't count because no-one saw you eat it....

You: There's not really enough left to share with husband/wife/kids/ flatmate, so I might as well finish it off.

Inner Child: Ooops, where did it all go?? Ooooh look, a puppy!!

Oh dear... If you'd had just one single Personal Policy in place, this disaster could've been averted! Despite the somewhat unruly nature of small children and your Inner Child, they really do respond extremely well to boundaries and rules, once they know what they are.

The WHEN/THEN Formula

So, let me show you an example of a very simple 3-part Supermarket Personal Policy that would have been the perfect foil in this situation:

WHEN I go to the Supermarket, THEN I...

...have a healthy snack beforehand.

...make a list and only buy what's on that list.

...do not venture down the confectionary aisle.

Actually, do you know what? Let's make this even simpler and distil it down into a single sentence:

WHEN I go to the Supermarket, THEN I...

...make a list and only buy what's on that list

That's it!!

I know it seems incredibly uncomplicated, but we humans have a habit of making things more difficult than they really are. Of course this Supermarket Personal Policy will require the tiniest little bit of preparation:

1) Decide what it is you're actually going to the Supermarket for.

2) Write a list.

Pretty easy, right?

Using the WHEN/THEN formula is a super-simple way to create your Personal Policies and help eliminate Decision Fatigue. Whether you're at home or out at an event, your Personal Policies will ensure you make the right choice without even thinking about it.

Now you know how easy it is, are you ready to create your own? I'll start you off with a few of my own Personal Polices:

WHEN I finish dinner at home, THEN I...

...have a cup of herbal tea to signify the end of the meal

WHEN I need an energy boost, THEN I...

...have a glass of water or a chat with a fun friend

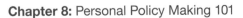

WHEN I am out and about, THEN I...

...always have a healthy snack (nuts or a protein bar) and a bottle of water with me

Your turn! Here are some hints for each category that will help you with your "**THEN I...**" statements:

I Need Energy!

Quite often, you're actually dehydrated and water is what you really need. Simply moving your body gets the blood pumping and is also an excellent tactic. If you truly are hungry, nuts, fruit, cheese, veggies & dip – the list goes on – are much better options, because they provide sustainable energy – not that horrendous sugar high-crash-high cycle.

It's a Habit

Create new habits e.g. have a glass of water, cup of tea or a square of dark chocolate (anything over 80% cacao is a good choice) after dinner. Perhaps brush your teeth or have a piece of gum straight after a meal when you would normally reach for something sweet. The next chapter really picks apart this 'habit' business and will help you analyse and short-circuit your automatic behaviours.

Mindlessness

Usually, this happens when you're being distracted by something else – most likely the television or computer screen. If you want to indulge, make it a Personal Policy to only take a small serve to the screen with you, wrapping the rest of it up and storing it away.

Peer Pressure

Birthday cake is a classic example, but there are plenty of other situations where there's pressure to consume sugar. We talked about a few ways to celebrate without sugar in the last chapter – be creative and dream up some more ideas that are unique and memorable. Isn't that what celebrating is really all about?

Availability – It's just there!

At home, it's very simple: have a Personal Policy of "I don't keep sugar at my house"! At work, it might be a little more difficult, but there are some very effective (and fun!) techniques outlined in Chapter 14 that you can implement.

WHEN I _____

THEN I _____

WHEN I _____

THEN I _____

WHEN I _____

THEN I _____

WHEN I _____

THEN I _____

WHEN I _____

THEN I _____

Bonus Smart Tip

I have a Personal Policy of never watching news programmes or reading news-only websites. If a massive, earth-shattering event happens, I'm pretty sure I'll hear about it somehow! I can then decide for myself if I want to go and find out more. The reason? I don't want someone else deciding for me what kind of world we live in. If I went by what's on the news, I would believe that the globe is a horrible place full of murder, kidnappings, bombings and political unrest. This can have a HUGE effect on your psyche, even if you don't realise it consciously. All those negative images lead to a totally defeatist attitude towards the future, which affects your behaviour in the now. Your subconscious will have even more "evidence" to sabotage you and it will start asking questions like:

- Why bother eating healthily if you're just going to be blown up by an extremist next time you go to the coffee shop?

- Who cares if you get diabetes or kidney failure? The world will probably end before then!

- You're going to die young from breathing in all that pollution anyway, so what difference does it make if you poison your body with sugar?

Wow – what a Negative Nancy your subconscious really is! But cut it some slack and remember, all it wants to do is protect you and keep you safe. It prepares for the worst possible situation, even if the probability of it actually happening to you is extremely unlikely. Watching the news just gives your already over-imaginative subconscious even more negative scenarios to play out and worry about.

If you currently do watch the news, just go without it for one week. I promise you won't miss it at all and I guarantee you'll feel a whole lot better!

CHAPTER 9

THE TAO OF HABITS

"A change in bad habits leads to a change in life."

— Jenny Craig

CHAPTER 9

THE TAO OF HABITS

"A habit is just an automatic action you've forgotten to take control of."
— Tara Mitchell

Many of us try to change our "bad" habits by making New Year's Resolutions which, by the way, is the single most ineffective way to actually change! I'll explain exactly why later on, but in the meantime, ask yourself this:

How can a statement made (most likely in an intoxicated state!) late at night on an arbitrary day that delineates the end of a human year can undo months and sometimes years of a certain behaviour?

The answer: It can't!

You know it, I know it, every gym and weight-loss club knows it, yet their sign-ups still rocket up every year in January… and the clubs are deserted again before the end of February. Why is this? Well, here's a clue: If you had to guess, how much uninterrupted effort do you think it would take to become another person? When I say 'another person', I don't mean how much plastic surgery would it take you to end up looking like Angelina Jolie or Brad Pitt! I mean a 'morning person' or a 'gym person' or a 'non-smoking person' if you aren't one already. There are some mythical numbers floating around…

- 7 days

- 21 days

- 30 days

Interesting how these correlate with sales pitches for various products, isn't it? Like:

- 7 Days to Drop a Dress Size!

- 21 Days to A New You!

- 30 Day Beach Body Challenge!

According to one study, it actually takes 66 (that's right SIXTY-SIX!) days before any kind of new behaviour becomes automatic – or a true habit. That means you're looking at over two whole months before you "just go" to the gym as part of your daily routine. That's without ANY disruptions – getting sick, pulling a muscle or missing a session (that turns into three or four or five or six sessions) that turns you into a couch potato again. Because we all believe we can magically become someone else in "30 days or less", when it gets to mid-February and things haven't transformed dramatically, we lose heart and give up.

The old habits that you snap back to are formed by long stretches of repetition, etched into your brain thanks to years of practice. Your brain just loves mindless, repetitive habits because they're highly efficient. Shifting into autopilot, generating patterns and sequences makes it simple for the brain to create shortcuts and routines. This makes it quicker and easier to get through your day using the least amount of brainpower possible.

Why is this important? Well, think about learning to tie your shoelaces for the first time. Remember how long it took when you were small? Think back and remember…

…the intense concentration it took to grasp the concept.

…the frustration when you couldn't quite get it.

...the annoyance you felt when you had to give up and ask for help.

...the time you spent practising over and over and over again.

...the feeling of pride and accomplishment when you finally got it right!

Can you imagine if every skill you have now required the same effort as when you were first learning it? How on earth would you get through the day if you had to expend as much energy on:

...getting dressed.

...making breakfast.

...brushing your teeth.

...locking the doors of your house.

...driving.

...writing.

...typing.

...doing laundry.

...etc.

...etc.

...etc.

That roller coaster of mental effort and emotions is extremely taxing, so your brain eventually works out little routines to make things like tying your shoelaces easy. Years later, you barely have to think about it. What happens now if your shoelace comes undone when you're walking? I bet you can just bend down, tie it back up again in less than

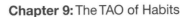

ten seconds, hardly breaking stride and moving on with your life. If I asked you about the last time you had to tie your shoelace, would you even recall the event? Well, maybe – if you didn't tie it up tight, it came loose and you stepped on it, falling flat on your face. I'm guessing you'd remember that! But usually it requires so little brainpower, it wouldn't even register on your radar.

This is how and why habits are created and for the most part, they're actually very useful. Habits free your brain up to concentrate on more complex tasks or to learn new things. They can be helpful or not so helpful – to decide which it is, ask yourself this question:

How is this habit serving me?

Any dentist would agree that a twice-daily teeth-brushing habit is serving you very well.

The six-teaspoons-sugar-in-your-morning-coffee habit? Not so much!

The TAO of Habits

There are plenty of studies on habits, how to break bad ones and create new good ones. Articles and books on the subject abound, especially around late December and early January! People have completed PhDs and dissertations on the subject and you can go on courses or retreats to help you with them. But what I've discovered is that all you need to do is become aware of your habit and track its path – then can you work out exactly what you need to do to change it.

I've created a very simple 3-Step method for you to identify why certain things are habitual for you and a really easy way to change them. I promise it will be a lot quicker than 66 days!

There are 3 phases to every habit, or what I like to call the TAO of Habits:

Trigger

Action

Outcome

I felt very pleased when I realised that this acronym is also a Chinese concept signifying "path" or "route". Habits are a path your brain has created and by using the TAO Method, you can create a brand new path and a brand new habit. What's really cool about this is that the Chinese philosophy of TAO is not about "getting" a concept intellectually, it's about actually living an experience to understand it. In consciously identifying your Triggers, then the current Actions and Outcomes you use in response and switching them out for better ones, you're creating a more enlightened and empowered you.

But that's enough philosophising for now! Let's take a closer look at some examples of the TAO Method in action. You're actually performing tens, sometimes hundreds of habitual actions in a day, mostly without a second thought. For example:

...the phone rings – Trigger

...you pick it up – Action

...you find out who's calling, satisfy your curiosity and talk to them – Outcome

As you can probably work out from reading the opening chapter, a very strong Trigger for me to seek out sugar was 'feeling tired'. One Action would then be to drink Coke and the Outcome would be for me to feel

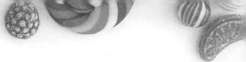

energised again… but only for a very short time. Because I made that link between drinking Coke and the positive feeling of being energised, it very quickly became a habit. In order to break that habit, what I had to do was associate drinking Coke with a negative feeling. I'll show you exactly how to do that in Chapter 12 – I know you're on the edge of your seat now!

Another Trigger for me used to be finishing dinner. Again, the Action would be to seek out something sugary as soon as I'd eaten my main meal, as I'd been trained from a young age that dinner always concluded with dessert. The Outcome was that I felt that dinner was 'finished'.

If you had a childhood like mine where ice-cream was often served after dinner, you might also have experienced this phenomenon: trying to give up dessert as an adult left you roaming the house in the evening, not really sure what was missing, but finally settling when you had something sweet. That's when the psychological signal was activated to tell you the evening meal was actually over and done with. In order to break this habit, I had to use a different technique. I needed to substitute in something else to tell my brain that dinner was finished. By creating the signal "a cup of tea means the end of dinner", it stopped my subconscious looking for something sweet.

In the above two examples, most people would have tried the advice to just "quit" Coke or dessert by using Willpower. But you already know why that doesn't work! I'm sure you can already see how useful the TAO Method is in identifying what's really going on with your habitual sugar consumption.

I bet you're keen to try it out for yourself, so let's do it!

We're now going to build on the exercise we did in the previous chapter. Go ahead and read through those top five times you wrote down that you felt you "needed" sugar. You might already find that you no longer think of these situations as Triggers, or you might decide you'd like to use the TAO Method to change your reaction to them.

Below is some space to write down your five Triggers, the old Action you took and the Outcome. The Action is obviously going to be to seek out some kind of sugar, but what kind exactly is it?

…a doughnut at morning tea to bond with your co-workers?

…a chocolate bar for some energy at 3pm?

…ice-cream after dinner?

I also want you to really think deeply about what the Outcome truly is for you. Is it…

…acceptance from your tribe?

…feeling rewarded?

…an escape or distraction? From what exactly?

…an indulgence?

…the signal for the end of a meal?

The last part of the exercise is to uncover the Emotions you experience immediately after the Outcome is met. Think back to the last time you responded to each of your Triggers. Remember…

…where you were

…who you were with

…what sounds you could hear

…what you were wearing

…how you were feeling

…why you chose the Action you did

Then ask yourself this question:

When you took the old Action you used to take in response to your Trigger, what feelings did you experience just after the Outcome?

Now, I'm not psychic or anything, but I'm absolutely certain whatever feelings you had after scoffing too much sugar to achieve your Outcome weren't good – which is why you want to change it, yes? To show you exactly what I mean, I'll use the two examples of my previous habits:

- **Trigger:** *Finishing Dinner.*

- **Action (old):** *Seek out and eat something sweet – usually ice-cream or milk chocolate.*

- **Outcome:** *Dinner is "finished" in my mind.*

- **Post-Outcome Feeling:** *Guilty for overeating, as I was already full from dinner.*

  Silly for eating ice-cream just before bedtime. The sugar-rush means I won't sleep well.

  Dumb - I should know better!

- **Trigger:** *Feeling tired or lethargic.*

- **Action (old):** *Drink two cans of Coke.*

- **Outcome:** *Energy!*

- **Post-Outcome Feelings:** *Worried about the effect of Coke on my teeth.*

   Guilty for spoiling all the hard work and money that went into my teeth (orthodontics).

   Uneasy about the sugar-crash I knew was coming and how I would cope with it.

Your turn! Here's the space for you to conduct your very own TAO Method analysis:

Trigger_____

Action (Old) _____

Outcome _____

Post-Outcome Feelings_____

_____

_____

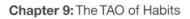

Trigger_____

Action (Old) _____

Outcome _____

Post-Outcome Feelings _____

_____

_____

Trigger_____

Action (Old) _____

Outcome _____

Post-Outcome Feelings _____

_____

_____

Trigger_____

Action (Old) _____

Outcome _____

Post-Outcome Feelings_____

_____

_____

Trigger_____

Action (Old) _____

Outcome _____

Post-Outcome Feelings_____

_____

_____

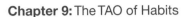

Mindfulness and honesty are the keys to this method. Be really truthful with yourself about what you feel after a sugar-binge in reaction to one of your Triggers. This will help you become aware of the real effects sugar has on you, after the initial rush has dropped off.

Now comes the best part! Remember how I said that New Year's Resolutions are the single most ineffective way to break a habit? Do you want to know what the MOST effective way is? Of course you do! Here's The Secret:

Replace the old Action that doesn't serve you with a new positive Action.

Hang on, wait a minute now. I don't have to slog it out using Willpower or sheer force for 66 days? That's all –just replace the old Action with a shiny new Action?

Yep – that's all!

I know this might sound pretty simple (are you starting to notice a pattern here?!) but when you've tried to break habits before, have you actually sat down and analysed them like you did above? I'm guessing perhaps not.

So of course your next step is to consciously choose a positive Action to your Trigger which not only meets your Outcome, but leaves you feeling great! Again, I'll show you mine (but only if you promise to show me yours!):

- **Trigger:** *Finishing Dinner.*

- **New Positive Action:** *Have a cup of herbal tea in a fancy glass.*

- **Outcome:** *Dinner is "finished" in my mind.*

- **Post-Outcome Feeling:** *Calm from the relaxing ritual of making and sipping tea.*

  Content that I will be able to sleep well.

  Happy I am looking after my body, hydrating it and adding antioxidants.

- **Trigger:** *Feeling tired or lethargic.*

- **New Positive Action:** *Work out what I really need – water, a healthy snack or maybe just cheering up!*

- **Outcome:** *Sustained energy.*

- **Post-Outcome Feelings:** *Pleased I'm looking after my body, especially my teeth!*

  Calm, knowing there won't be any sugar-rush-crash cycle to deal with.

  Confident I'm doing the best thing for my health.

OK - now it's over to you. What I'd love for you to do is create some really positive new Actions for your five Triggers and write them down below. You may not face some of your Triggers for a while yet, so for now, just image how good you'll feel when you respond with your new Actions! Run through the situation in your mind and step through exactly what you're going to do next time.

When next time comes around, take note of all those great feelings you get from taking your positive Action. Come back here and write them down – you'll be so proud of yourself and how far you've come (and so will I!).

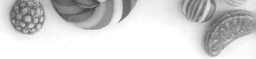

Trigger_____

New Positive Action _____

Outcome _____

Post-Outcome Feelings _____

_____

_____

Trigger_____

New Positive Action _____

Outcome _____

Post-Outcome Feelings _____

_____

_____

Trigger_____

New Positive Action _____

Outcome _____

Post-Outcome Feelings _____

_____

_____

Trigger_____

New Positive Action _____

Outcome _____

Post-Outcome Feelings _____

_____

_____

Trigger_____

New Positive Action _____

Outcome _____

Post-Outcome Feelings_____

_____

_____

How good do you feel??!!

CHAPTER 10

MANAGE YOUR MIND...
MINDFULLY!

"Mind is a flexible mirror, adjust it, to see a better world."

— Amit Ray

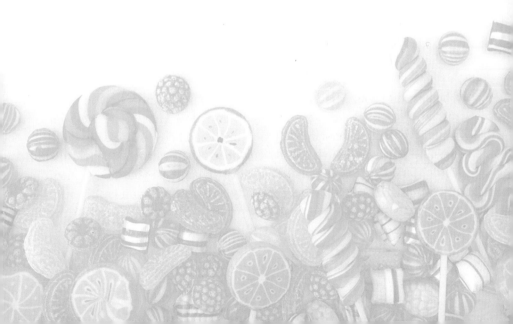

CHAPTER 10

MANAGE YOUR MIND...MINDFULLY!

"Paying attention creates bigger dividends than any other kind of investment!"
— Tara Mitchell

You've heard the term Mindfulness bandied about in the media a lot lately, but there seems to be a fair bit of confusion about what it actually means. Most people seem to think Mindfulness takes a huge amount of Willpower (and we all know how well that works!) and the discipline of a Tibetan monk. Complete control of your thoughts leads to the total emptiness of your mind and is the singular path to reach true Nirvana. You might wish to take this route if your quest is supreme self-enlightenment, however most of us really just want to get through the day in one piece!

Mindfulness actually not complicated at all and, at its core, is really very straightforward; in a nutshell, it's being aware of and observing **You**, in the moment, right now.

It really is that simple.

The best bit about Mindfulness is that you already know how to think this way – no orange robes required! How do I know that? Well, on some level, you understand that your mind and body are actually quite separate things, although closely entwined. The companies behind the Dirty Marketing Tricks want you believe you are just your body – how else would they get you to feel so guilty about the way you look?

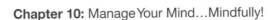

When you think about it, it's actually quite bizarre to think that unless we have a perfect body, we can't be a perfect friend/partner/sibling/parent/employee. But to be a great person, all you really have to do is be mindful about how you speak and act towards others. This has nothing at all to do with your body – it all happens in your mind!

We also think that the evil twin of Mindfulness is Mindlessness – and it's this Mindlessness that causes us to:

…thoughtlessly grab a chocolate bar at 3pm.

…automatically serve ourselves sweets after dinner without thinking.

…hoover up a whole bag of Jaffas at the movies.

…finish off the whole tub of ice-cream without even realising.

I don't believe Mindlessness is inherently evil – I actually think you can make friends with Mindlessness so it's working WITH you, rather than against you! Why not flip the switch so your mindless choices are the best choices, and you really have to think about the bad choices?

So, how do we do this? Well, first we need to understand and accept the separation between mind and body. Marketers have been conditioning you for years to think that you are your body, but here's a nifty question which proves that you're actually immune to their brainwashing:

If you were to break your arm (heaven forbid!), would you say:

a) "My arm is broken!"

or

b) "I am broken!" ?

Unless you're feeling a little melodramatic (and that's perfectly OK if you are, we all do sometimes!) I'm pretty sure you would've answered a). You probably know (even if you haven't actually experienced it) that a broken arm isn't much fun and it really hurts – which might stop you thinking straight for a while! There are definitely some other effects a broken arm has on your mind – perhaps you might avoid repeating the activity that broke your arm (unless you're a teenaged boy!) or develop a particular attitude towards hospitals, depending on how you were cared for.

But in the end, a broken arm doesn't define you or how you think. A broken arm doesn't make you any less smart or significantly alter your core values about life, nor does it become part of your identity. Once the cast is off and you're fully recovered, you don't go about introducing yourself at dinner parties by saying "Hi, I'm Sally and I am a broken arm". Of course, it will come up in conversation at times, but you recognise that it's something that happened and had a relatively fleeting effect on your life, although it might not have seemed fleeting at the time.

This is the basis of how Mindfulness works – recognising and observing what's happening, but being conscious that it doesn't affect your whole being, nor devastate your future.

So guess what else this means? Not only are You not your body, You are not your emotions! Emotions are fleeting in exactly the same way as a broken arm is, even though they might feel like they totally consume you at the time. They do not form your identity and they are not part of your value system. Like the broken arm example, you don't go around introducing yourself by saying "Hi, I'm Sally and I am anxious"! Emotions are something you can choose to DO, not BE in any given situation – yes that's right, you CAN choose not to be angry at someone! Don't believe me? Stay tuned – I'll give you a great example of how I do it in the next chapter!

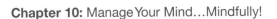

Even though we're aware that we do actually have a choice in every situation, emotions can sometimes lead us to actions we regret later. Have you ever shouted at someone in anger, snarled at someone in fear or eaten a whole tub of ice-cream in sadness and wished you hadn't? You know that the emotion has a lot to do with your attraction to sugar, but why should you let something so fleeting have such control over your long-term health?

We seem to think that managing emotions is a massive challenge, but would you like to know a way to work with those emotions so they don't totally overtake your rational thinking? Here's an approach I've discovered that works really well for me, and I'm pretty sure it will work for you too:

When you have a sugar "craving", identify the emotion you're feeling and name it out loud.

But what's the point of naming the emotion, you might ask – I know when I'm feeling sad! It's readily important to do this because naming something helps you manage and control it. Have you ever had a pet dog or cat? What's the very first thing you do? You give it a name, right? Animals may not speak English, but they do respond to their name and can be trained to come when you call them. There's also massive power in a name – how often have you tuned out a conversation in the background, but suddenly sat up and taken notice when your name is mentioned?

Even better, when you acknowledge an emotion, it makes it easier to make a conscious decision about what you'd like instead. I don't believe in masking emotions or denying they exist – they're part of being human after all! In detaching the emotion from You, it's so much easier to deal with it logically, rather than letting your Lizard Brain take control. Truly being in the moment can help you see what other choices you have, rather than panicking and reacting irrationally.

It's really easy to get started too. All you have to do is become conscious of your decisions throughout the day, then ask a very simple question. This will alert you to where your actions have become embedded and automatic. Then you can establish what emotion is underlying your choice. This works equally well for good habits, as well as those you've decided are "bad" and you want out of your life. Identifying what drives you to make good decisions can also help you shift your bad habits. This is a really effective process – I find it's worthwhile to pay attention to even the smallest decisions you make in the course of a day. Any time you think consciously about a typical automatic behaviour, you increase focus on your actions, which alerts you to the fact you can choose to do something different.

Oh, I suppose I should let you know what the "very simple question" is! OK, when you catch yourself in an automatic behaviour, just ask:

"Why am I doing this?"

Maybe you're asking…

"Why am I eating sugary cereal in the morning?"

"Why am I having 2 sugars in my coffee?"

"Why am I saying yes to dessert?"

"Why am I eating chocolate at 3pm?"

"Why am I seeing the bottom of a family-sized tub of ice-cream?"

You may be able to answer identify an obvious emotion straight away. But sometimes, especially if your subconscious is anything like mine, it will come back with a smart-arse response like "Because I want to!!". In this case, you just reassure your Inner Child that it's not in trouble, but you would like to know what's going on because you care very much. You can then dig deeper by asking this question:

"And why is that important?"

You might need to ask this question a couple more times, but it won't take long before you uncover the real reason behind the choice. Let me give you a personal example of when I asked this question of myself:

"Why am I having ice-cream for breakfast?"

Besides the snappy "Because I want to!!" response, I also got:

"Because dairy is good for your bones."

Then I continued on and asked the second question a couple of times, and this is what I uncovered:

…and why is that important?

"Because I don't want to get osteoporosis."

…and why is that important?

"Because I don't want to lose my independence when I get older."

…and why is that important?

"Because relying 100% on other people to look after me is really scary!"

Interesting… on the surface, I was justifying my breakfast ice-cream habit by claiming it was good for me, when really I was scared of the consequences of not consuming dairy. So it was fear that was the driver and if you're fearful, you become an easy target for marketers. I had been brainwashed to believe dairy was the only way to get strong bones, which of course is not true. You know that fear is a very powerful motivator and you also know that knowledge is the antidote to fear. Once I worked this out, it became very easy for me to establish much better habits.

A word of warning when using this line of questioning – this is the only time I want you to ask "Why…?". Questions can be incredibly energetic tools when used correctly, but "Why…?" questions can lead to a depressing downward spiral. I'll reveal why that is (pun intended!) and also show you how to harness their awesome power for good in Chapter 13.

Now that you know how to find the emotion behind your Mindless behaviour, it's time we talked about how to reprogram your reaction to it.

THE NRC Technique to Reprogramming Emotional Reactions

Here's my really simple 3-Step NRC Technique you can use to reprogram your reaction to emotions:

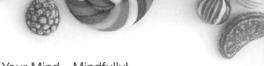

NAME   **RELEASE**   **CHOOSE**

It won't be long before you're doing this automatically, but of course you'll need a bit of practice to begin with, as with anything new. Let's start with an example…

Step 1) NAME The Emotion Out Loud:

Catch yourself when you feel a sugar craving and figure out exactly what it is you're feeling. If it's sadness, for example, rather than saying:

"I feel sad"

Say:

"There is sadness there."

OK, great start – we've identified what the emotion is here. The next step is to identify what your usual reaction is. Perhaps this is where you'd normally reach for chocolate to cheer yourself up? Recognise and accept this is what you might have done in the past and that's totally OK. You can't alter your history, and beating yourself up about it definitely won't change it! But what you CAN do is change the way you think about it, as well as make a conscious choice to do something better in the future.

Step 2) RELEASE Your Past Reaction to the Emotion:

Acknowledge your past reaction, write it down and release it by saying it out loud. For example:

"This is where I used to eat a family block of chocolate, which I used to think would help me deal with sadness. Now I know better and I release sadness easily and effortlessly."

Appreciate that you did your best in the past, but now you know chocolate won't fix the feeling. In fact, you now know that demolishing a whole block of chocolate will actually make you feel WORSE! You now have a whole world of choices that are more empowering and will serve you better.

Step 3) CHOOSE A Better Option:

What would serve you better than eating a block of chocolate when you identify sadness in your life?

Write down a list.

Here are some ideas:

- Watch a funny video.

- Sniff essential oils (citrus scents & lavender are great choices).

- Look through photos of family or your last holiday.

- Call a friend.

- Take a walk around the block.

- Write in your journal.

- Count your blessings.

- Remember a great achievement, however small – even winning a ribbon at school sports day!

- Meditate.

- Listen to an upbeat song.

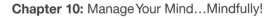

Once you have your list, decide which one you will do next time you identify sadness in your life. The first time you may have to consciously remember to do it, but very soon you won't even need to think about it. It will become a Mindless choice that you don't have to expend any energy on.

Here's some space to write down three of your own 3-Step NCR Plans:

1) NAME the Emotion _____

2) RELEASE the Emotion. *"This is where I used to* _____

_____

_____ *"*

"Now I know better and I can release _____ *easily and effortlessly."*

List your Better Options:

_____

_____

_____

3) CHOOSE Your Better Option: _____

1) NAME the Emotion _____

2) RELEASE the Emotion. *"This is where I used to* _____

_____

_____ *"*

"Now I know better and I can release _____
easily and effortlessly."

List your Better Options:

_____

_____

_____

_____

3) CHOOSE Your Better Option: _____

_____

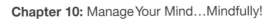

1) NAME the Emotion _____

2) RELEASE the Emotion. *"This is where I used to* _____

_____

_____ *"*

"Now I know better and I can release _____
easily and effortlessly."

List your Better Options:

_____

_____

_____

_____

3) CHOOSE Your Better Option: _____

_____

Hey, guess what? We just reduced your Decision Fatigue again – great work!

The Shortcut Method

Sometimes you find yourself in a situation where an emotion comes up that you hadn't planned out an NRC response to. That's OK, I've been there too and I've got your back! Here's the short-circuit version of the NRC Method you can use on the fly to disconnect yourself from an emotion.

Remember how we replaced "I feel sad" with "There is sadness there"? You also remember that emotions are something we choose to DO, not BE? We are not our emotions, just like we are not our bodies. So next time you catch yourself unexpectedly feeling sad for example, say this:

"I am doing Sadness right now."

Notice the action verb "doing" in that sentence? This implies that we are taking a specific action right now and guess what? Humans don't do any kind of action indefinitely (even ones we really enjoy!) so this tells your brain that the action has an end point. We're still acknowledging the emotion, which is important to do, but we know that it won't go on forever. We are free to choose something else if we want. Your brain will already be thinking ahead to what the next activity will be!

CHAPTER 11

INNER TALK

"Do you kiss your mother with that mouth?"

— Wayne Campbell

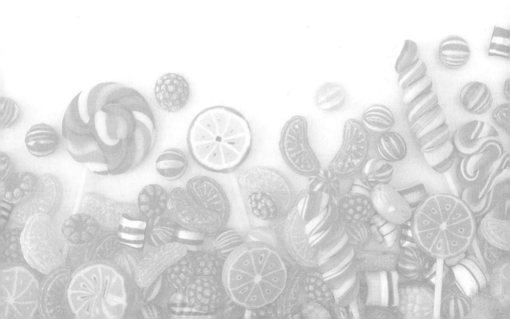

CHAPTER 11

INNER TALK

"Take control of the voice inside your head... before somebody else does!"
— Tara Mitchell

Do you talk to yourself in your head? It's OK – everyone does it, some of us even do it out loud! But let me ask you this:

How do you talk to yourself?

Is it positive and encouraging? Or does it go more like this if you mindlessly scoff an entire family tub of ice-cream:

"You bloody idiot, I can't believe you did that – again! You're always doing dumb things like that! What's wrong with you? Can't you get anything right? Don't you have any self-control?"

Do you get angry and worked up, berating yourself for the simplest things and every minor slip-up? Are you always asking yourself why or how you could do such a stupid thing? Every time you do this, you're kicking the puppy that is your Inner Child (sorry for that image, but you are!) Your Inner Child is not just a figment of New-Age mysticism, although the term can conjure up images of long-haired hippies clad in flowing robes of purple tie-dye (or is that just me??!).

The Inner Child is within every one of us and is just like Peter Pan – it never grows up, it stays around six or seven years old. Things start making a whole lot more sense when you understand your subconscious is this age. Think about the true impulse you have when no-one else is around:

- When you see a pile of freshly-raked leaves in autumn, are you just dying to take a running jump at it, kicking up leaves in the air and squealing with delight?

- Do you sometimes have an irresistible urge to run shopping trolley races up and down the Supermarket aisles?

- Would you abandon your spreadsheets and engage in office chair races if you were left unsupervised for the afternoon?

These windows into the spontaneous nature of how you'd act if no-one was watching are the joyous and fun side of your Inner Child.

But, as anyone who's had experience with small children knows, a gale of laughter can turn into a howling tantrum in a split second when something is denied them. It's exactly the same with your Inner Child. If you deny them sweets, ice-cream, doughnuts or whatever it is they want, there's gonna be trouble! If you keep speaking to your Inner Child angrily, they'll keep chucking tantrums and will need to be placated.

How many times have you seen a small child lose their mind in the Supermarket aisle because they can't have the lollies, biscuits or toy they wanted? Then, it seems, the distraction technique is the only option "I'll take you for ice-cream/buy you a lollypop afterwards if you behave!" Your Inner Child is just the same. You upset them, they need to be placated. What we really want is to avoid upsetting them in the first place! Let me show you how easy this is – there's pretty much just one simple rule to live by:

Speak to yourself like you would a six-year-old child.

What?

Seems a bit silly, but go with me on this one!

Imagine you have a small child visiting. If they dropped their drink on the floor, you'd never speak to them harshly, like you did to yourself when you ate too much ice-cream (at least, I hope you wouldn't!!) I imagine you'd say something much kinder and more encouraging:

"Oops-a-daisy! Next time we'll hold onto our cup a bit tighter and keep our eyes faced towards where we're walking, won't we?"

Or words to that effect. When you speak encouragingly to your Inner Child, they are less likely to throw a tantrum and demand a "treat" as a pacifier. Talking to yourself like a small child that's visiting you might make you feel a little silly at first, but I guarantee you'll feel lighter, more whimsical and happier overall.

Be Kind to Yourself

Ever heard the saying "You catch more flies with honey than vinegar"? If you haven't, now is a great time to start living by it! Not only is it more likely to get you what you want when dealing with other people, you're far more likely to tame your Inner Child by being encouraging rather than critical.

Interestingly, major hotel chains have moved away from asking guests to report staff doing the wrong thing to "catching" them doing their best. Time and again, it's been proven that catching someone doing something RIGHT and ENcouraging the behaviour is far more effective than catching someone doing something WRONG and DIScouraging (or "correcting") the behaviour. Everyone needs something to aim for – give anyone a target, and they'll do their best to hit it. It's what every sport on the planet is based on!

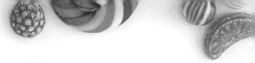

Humans inherently want to be rewarded for good behaviour and to celebrate their successes. Every single workplace cited as the best in the world to work for has a culture of highlighting success. It encourages innovative thinking, length of service, and employees will "go the extra mile" when they know they'll be recognised for it. Do this for yourself – make sure to give yourself a little mental high-five or pat on the pack (whatever suits your personal style) when you know you done good kid! Your Inner Child will respond, feeling very proud and wanting to build on that behaviour.

Keep an 'ENcouragement list' of the times you catch yourself doing something good and describe how it made you feel. You'll see shortly why it's such a good idea to actually write these down, so you can refer back later. The small things make the biggest difference and they're the easiest to achieve, so don't worry if you haven't run a marathon today! It can be something as simple as:

"I had an apple and almond butter for afternoon tea today instead of a chocolate bar. I felt so much better not having a sugar-crash afterwards and, I have to admit, I feel a little bit virtuous. I like this feeling!"

Here's some space for you to keep your ENcouragement list:

_____

_____

_____

_____

_____

_____

_____

_____

_____

_____

_____

_____

Writing these down is concrete proof that you are actually pretty awesome – and doesn't that sound like something that might make you feel better when you look back and read it again? Just the tiniest boost to your confidence can make all the difference!

Reframing

Now, being kind to yourself is not only about recognising when you've done well, but knowing that slipping up is not the end of the world. Quite often, one tiny misstep on our path can have us spiralling down at the speed of light.

> "Oh, %#@&!!! I ate one chocolate biscuit whilst I was supposed to be on my very strict diet... I'VE FAILED MISERABLY – I MIGHT AS WELL EAT THE WHOLE PACKET NOW, PLUS A TUB OF ICE-CREAM AND TWO FAMILY BLOCKS OF CHOCOLATE TO CONSOLE MYSELF. Boo hoo, woe is me..."

Sound familiar? You already know that diets don't work, but being really harsh and uncompromising on yourself will send you off the rails faster than you can say "Never-ending packet of Double-coat Tim Tams"! So how do we turn this slippery slope to misery into super-happy fun times?

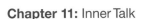

We use what's known as Reframing, which is kind of like seeking out the silver lining, to use a cliché, but much more potent.

Reframing is such a great technique, because it can change the entire meaning you take from a situation. And the best bit? We can make it so much fun that it seems like a game, but in reality you're reprogramming your neural pathways. Longer term, this means you can train yourself to react exactly how you want to, rather than with high emotion which, as you know, you often regret later. After practising this for a while, you'll be able to turn yourself from fuming with anger to dissolving into gales of laughter within seconds. How do I know this? Because I've done it and I know you can too! Let me share with you my first experience of Reframing in a formal setting.

We were asked to think of something that had recently made us really angry and then Reframe it. I immediately remembered a situation where I'd been driving down the highway in peak hour traffic. Suddenly, some maniac in a red sports car comes speeding out of nowhere, weaving in and out of traffic, cutting other cars off and barely making it though gaps with millimetres to spare. My reaction was to see red!!

"What a bloody idiot!! Doesn't he know how dangerously he's driving?? He's putting everyone on the road at risk, just so he can show off his stupid mid-life crisis car - what a #@^$!!!!"

Even just recalling the situation made me so angry! So how on earth did I reframe this situation so I was killing myself laughing? Here's what I came up with:

It's Administrative Professionals Day today and, just like the past five years, this horrible boss has forgotten. Every other P.A. in the office gets flowers and treated to lunch, but this guy's P.A. has spent the morning being screamed at for messing up a dinner reservation. It was supposed to be for a clandestine meeting with the mistress, but the P.A. accidentally sent the invite to the wife. After years of putting up with his temper tantrums and abuse, she's finally decided to hand in her resignation. To soften the blow, she hands him his favourite mocha skim cappuccino with EXACTLY 1 centimetre of froth and the precise amount of chocolate… loaded with fast-acting laxatives. He's just read though the letter when the phone rings – it's the police telling him his jealous not-so-secret mistress is threatening to set his house on fire and is exchanging blows with his wife out the front. He slams down the rest of his coffee and jumps into his red sports car, speeding back home before his entire life goes up in smoke. He's only a few minutes into his hour drive home on the freeway when suddenly, he gets an extreme gurgling sensation in his lower belly…

I know it's not nice to laugh at others' misfortunes, but as long as you're not inflicting the damage yourself, I think it's perfectly OK to use your imagination to your advantage! So I guess you're wondering how this silly story can help you Outsmart Sugar? I'm pretty sure you can think of some situations where viewing it from another perspective would serve you better.

Instead of thinking of sugar as a reward, Reframe it to what it really is: a poor substitute for real food and nourishment. You might want to take a look back to Chapter 3 "What Sugar Really Does to You…" to remind yourself of the real effects sugar has on you once the rush wears off.

The Procrastination Method

This is a fun way of using procrastination to your advantage. If you're anything like me, you'll do whatever it takes NOT to finish certain tasks – sorting through your tax receipts, ironing, or maybe finish writing your book (trust me, all authors are master-level procrastinators!). Things that wouldn't normally be even remotely appealing, like scrubbing the bathroom tile grout or organising the kitchen cupboards, become compelling and urgent. Your inner talk probably goes something like this:

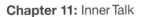

"Yeah, yeah – I know that needs to be done but… man, look at how untidy those cupboards are! That crockery and Tupperware isn't going to arrange itself neatly on its own! I can't live with it one second longer!"

Why not turn the idea of procrastination on its head and consider your sugar craving as something you can get to later? This gives your brain permission to acknowledge that you want it, which also satisfies your Inner Child. If you're even slightly good at procrastinating, you'll know that putting things off until "Sometime In The Future" means they often don't happen at all. Look at most people's spare rooms or garages! To use this to your advantage, when you desperately feel like sugar, just say to yourself:

"Yes, OK – you can have that a bit later."

Occupy yourself with something else in the meantime and nine times out of ten, you won't even remember what you wanted in the first place!

The Single Word That Will Change Your Destiny

I've saved the best until last for you here – this is my absolute favourite mind trick of all time, because it's so incredibly simple yet amazingly powerful. Technically, this is actually two words contracted – I'm taking just a pinch of poetic license here because it sounds much cooler than "the two contracted words that will change your destiny"! Forgive me? I hope so, because I promise this Jedi mind-trick will change your relationship with sugar (and any other food or drink that you want to end that bad-boyfriend-like attraction to) pretty much instantaneously.

Ready?

Swap out the word 'CAN'T' for 'DON'T'

That's it. Seriously.

How can such a simple change have such a dramatic effect? Let me demonstrate.

Try saying this out loud:

"I can't have a doughnut."

How did this make you feel? Sad? Frustrated? Disempowered?

Saying you "can't" do something implies that someone else is in charge and making decisions for you. You already know how your Inner Child is going to react to being told what to do, don't you?! "Can't" also indicates a state of lack or wanting, which is never a good emotional state to be in. As we saw in Chapter 3, humans react to scarcity by hoarding or consuming as much as they can. Every time you say "I can't have a chocolate bar" all your brain hears is "Oh my God – there's a world shortage of chocolate bars!! Quick, we must get ALL the chocolate bars before we die of chocolate deficiency!!"

Now try:

"I choose not to have a doughnut."

This is somewhat better, as it hands decision making firmly back to you. You (and your Inner Child) are in control, making all the grown-up decisions about what you will and won't eat. It's still not ideal though. What about the next time you're offered a doughnut?

And the next?

And the next?

What will you do then?

This just adds yet another choice to your day, which you can well do without.

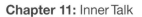

As you already know, your best course of action is to remove choice and reduce decision fatigue. Think you'll feel deprived and hard done by if you give yourself less choice? Research shows this isn't simply isn't so. Think of Henry Ford's famous comment to customers when choosing the colour of their Model T Ford:

"You can have any colour – so long as it's black."

Do you think potential motorists were upset about the lack of choice? Of course not!! They were so excited they no longer had to feed, water and clean up after their means of transport, the colour of the vehicle was totally immaterial.

Now try:

"I don't eat doughnuts."

Now again with a little conviction!

Maybe hold up your palm like you're saying "Stop!", even thrusting your hip out to the side if you're feeling a little sassy!

How did that feel?

Did you feel powerful and decisive?

In charge and at large?

When you say "I don't..." it's a very strong statement and actually forms part of your identity. Think about a vegetarian. They don't say, "I can't eat meat". They say "I DON'T eat meat". Not eating meat is very much part of their identity, it's categorically who they are and dictates how they interact with the rest of the world. Vegetarians don't choose steakhouse restaurants when they meet friends for dinner.

They don't keep pork chops and chicken breasts in their fridge at home. They don't eat meat just to "fit in" with whoever they're dining with.

Essential to your success with "I don't..." statements is CERTAINTY, just like vegetarians are absolutely certain they don't eat meat. When you are unequivocally sure of your intent, the outcome is inevitable!

Try out some "I don't..." statements for yourself here:

I don't _____

I don't _____

I don't _____

I don't _____

I don't _____

If you only use this one little trick out of everything you read in this book, make it this one. I guarantee this will give you the biggest bang for your buck – and all you need to do is change one little word! How good is that?!

CHAPTER 12

YEAH! TO MEH...

"The truth is that we can learn to condition our minds, bodies, and emotions to link pain or pleasure to whatever we choose. By changing what we link pain and pleasure to, we will instantly change our behaviours."

— Tony Robbins

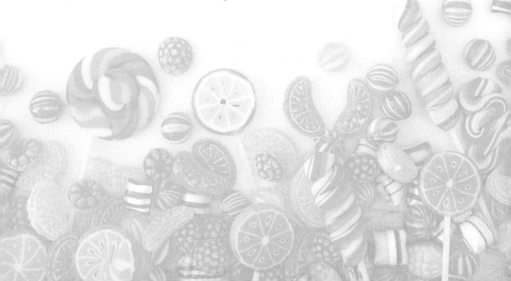

CHAPTER 12

YEAH! TO MEH...

"Harnessing your own subconscious is your Master Key to dismissing sugar easily and effortlessly!"
— Tara Mitchell

I know you've been waiting for this one! This is where it all started for me, my Ground Zero if you will. This process triggered my understanding of exactly how powerful the human brain is and started me on the path to writing this book. To be honest, it kinda freaked me out a little bit too, as it made me realise I held all the power. Not the sugar, not the Food Manufacturers, not the advertising companies, just little ol' me! This might be scary for you too, as it means taking total responsibility for your choices, but don't worry – it's really quite empowering and I'll be with you every step of the way.

As you know from reading the introduction, I learned how to flick the switch in my brain from what I thought was a hopeless "addiction" to sugar to finding sugar a mere curiosity. It might sound like utter sorcery to people who also think they are addicted to sugar, and I guess it is a kind of brain "magic". The truth of the matter is, it's actually very simple and it's probably already happened to you without you even knowing! What's amazing about this process is that it harnesses a perfectly normal human reaction to modify your subconscious reactions. No need to consciously think about it (thus reducing Decision Fatigue), and definitely no need for Willpower!

Now, I mentioned that I'm pretty sure you've experienced this phenomenon already in your life. How can I be so sure of this? Let me

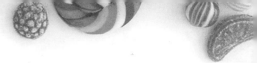

share with you a couple of events from my own life to see if anything similar has happened to you:

- The back yard of the house I grew up in had plenty of fruit trees, including a gorgeous dwarf orange tree. At three years old, I wasn't big enough to climb the other trees, but this little tree was less than two metres tall. When it bore a bumper crop of low-hanging, sweet juicy oranges, I did what any self-respecting unsupervised toddler would do and stuffed myself stupid! Dad still laughs when he tells the story of finding me in the back yard, completely drenched in orange juice, surrounded by chunks of orange peel, moaning and complaining about feeling sick in my tummy. I didn't touch oranges again until many years later.

- My trip to Thailand with a group of friends in my early twenties was exciting for many reasons. It was my first trip overseas with friends rather than family, experiencing the thrill of driving in another country and immersing myself completely in another culture. And of course the food! … until Coriander-gate. To this day, I'm still not entirely sure exactly what it was that made me so sick that I was bed-ridden for two days. I won't go into graphic detail, but I sure was a few kilos lighter after those two days! My friends had eaten at the same restaurant as I had, two of them even ordered the same meal – coriander stir-fried chicken – but, for some reason, I was the only one who got ill. All I could taste in my throat as that dinner made its way back up again (sorry, I did promise I wouldn't go into too much detail!) was the coriander. Days later, it was still there. It took me almost a decade to be able to face anything with coriander in it again.

If you've ever been so hungover the thought of consuming alcohol ever, ever again turns your stomach, you will also be familiar with this phenomenon. A hangover would normally be enough to stop you drinking again but, just like sugar, there are many positive associations with moderate consumption of alcohol, including bonding with your tribe and feeling relaxed.

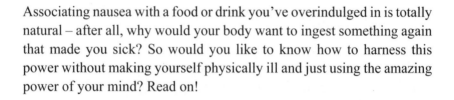

Associating nausea with a food or drink you've overindulged in is totally natural – after all, why would your body want to ingest something again that made you sick? So would you like to know how to harness this power without making yourself physically ill and just using the amazing power of your mind? Read on!

In my opinion, this is the most amazing piece of brain mastery there is, but you don't need to be a neuroscientist to get how this works. As you've probably guessed from my examples above, we basically take the reaction to sugary food or drink that you love (but want out of your life), and replace it with your reaction to something disgusting. Easy, right?

This process works best when you have a trained NLP coach work through this with you, as I did to rid me of my Coke "addiction". Go to **outsmartsugarnow.com** to check out my personalised coaching options I've designed just for you. In the meantime, let me share with you a method I've created you can follow easily on your own. I like to call it "Yeah! to Meh…". Where previously you would have said "Yeah!" (possibly even "Hell Yeah!") to a sugary treat, you'll now be able to say "Meh… not interested".

The single most important aspect of this technique is that you must truly want to dismiss this sugary Nemesis of yours out of your life. 100% commitment is required – nothing short of this will cut it I'm afraid. Are you willing and able to make this commitment to yourself and your health right now?

Are you sure?

100%?

Just to make certain, let's make a real commitment - sign this contract with yourself:

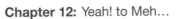

I _____

make a commitment to myself to dismiss sugar easily and effortlessly from my life.

Signed_____

Date _____

OK – you're in! So, how do we make this brain switch?

I need to warn you, I'm going to ask you to get a little bit uncomfortable – remember, getting outside your comfort zone is where change happens. To achieve real change, you need to stretch your comfort zone just enough so it becomes your new, expanded comfort zone. Massive change can be like stretching a rubber band too far – sometimes it breaks, but more often than not, it just snaps back to its original position.

This is why practically everyone who wins the Lotto jackpot ends up back exactly where they were pre-jackpot after around two years or so. As do most contestants on shows like the Biggest Loser. Without undertaking the proper inner work, will never match your outer world and (as you now know), your Amygdala will do everything in its power to make sure you stay in your comfort zone. Enough already, I hear you say – just show me how to do it!!

Decide on what it is you currently say "Yeah!" to without thinking and want to be able to shrug your shoulders and just say "Meh. No, thank you". Being really precise here is key. Just choosing "Cake" is generic and it's too confusing for your brain to cover all the different permutations of "Cake" that are available. Whatever it is you choose, we're going to name it your Nemesis.

It's absolutely imperative that you get specific on you Nemesis. And I do mean REALLY specific and absolutely clear on that thing you want to dismiss, easily and effortlessly. I know I'm repeating myself here, but it really is essential that you identify EXACTLY what you want out of your life. Just so we're clear, let me illustrate with an example:

You already know it was Coke that started me on this journey – it was my Nemesis for quite some time. Just deciding on 'soft drink' would have been far too general – it comes in bright yellow, brilliant orange, dark brown, light brown, cobalt blue, grassy green, raspberry red… OK, I think you get the picture! There's loads of variables with soft drink, as there is with sugar in general. So I had to get really specific and name my Nemesis "Coke".

So – what is it for you?

Is it cake? Specifically – what kind?

- Is it chocolate mud cake?

- Is it Tiramisu?

- Is it cheesecake?

Is it doughnuts? Seems specific enough, but which ones make you stuff your face like there's a world shortage of them?

- Chocolate iced doughnuts?

- Powdered sugar doughnuts?

- Hot cinnamon doughnuts?

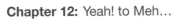

Perhaps chocolate is your Nemesis. Again, choose one specifically:

- A certain brand of dairy milk chocolate?

- A kind of chocolate bar?

- One particular boxed chocolate?

I cannot overemphasise the importance of getting specific for this to work – it will become very obvious why shortly!

If you're a little concerned that you're narrowing your options, just remember we can always come back and do this exercise again later on if you'd like to. But, interestingly, I find that people who fully commit to this exercise up front find they can flip that switch in their brain any time they want. They now find it easy to dismiss anything else they know isn't in their best interest.

So – write down what it is, very specifically, that you want to dismiss out of your life. Name your Nemesis!

_____

Focus on that thing, very closely. Close your eyes and think about it, feel it through your body and form a picture in your mind of you with your Nemesis. Imagine seeing it, picking it up, opening the wrapper or packet or tub and getting stuck in. Taste it, noticing how it makes you feel.

Write down below what you saw in your mind:

1) Is the picture you see in your mind black and white or colour?

_____

2) Is it close to you or far away?

_____

3) Is it bright or dim?

_____

4) Is it moving like a movie, or flat like a framed painting?

_____

5) Do you see yourself in the picture, or are you looking at the scene through your own eyes?

_____

Great, thank you for answering those questions. Ooooooh – do you smell popcorn??

No?

Sorry, must just be me! Let's move on to the next bit of the process.

OK, now I want you to choose something so disgusting that it turns your stomach just thinking about it. Here's the catch: it needs to look like or share some characteristics with your chosen Nemesis. This is why it's so important to be exactly specific. Again, if you chose "Cake", there's far too many variables to accurately match something revolting to it.

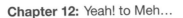

However, if you said "Chocolate Mud Cake", I don't think I need to let your imagination run too far to think of something dark brown, dense and gooey that would turn your stomach if you had to eat it!

Dream up the most Revolting Thing you can possibly think of. Make sure it's bad, REALLY BAD and that it's absolutely and truly foul and disgusting to you. Make a commitment to play full out here – I'll know if you haven't been playing hard enough, the test is coming up soon!

Now write that most disgusting thing down here, being as descriptive as you possibly can (don't worry, nobody's looking!). What is your Revolting Thing?

_____

_____

_____

I promised you a test – bet you didn't think it was going to be this soon though! I'll know pretty quickly if you've been genuinely creative by your answer to this question:

Would you eat that Revolting Thing if I paid you $100?

No? Good.

Would you eat that Revolting Thing if I gave you $50,000?

Still no? We're on the right track! Now the big question:

Would you eat that Revolting Thing if I gave you a MILLION DOLLARS?

Hmmmmmm, now you're thinking about it, aren't you?

If the answer's still no, you have chosen wisely. If the answer's yes –
it's time to get even more creative and venture into that dark corner of
your brain that you hide from polite company. You have to get down
and dirty, playing in the gutters of your mind for this to really, truly
work. The Million Dollar Test will uncover if your chosen thing is truly
disgusting enough to make an impact on your brain. Please forgive me if
you've just eaten, but here are some words to start you thinking:

- Poisonous
- Moulded
- Rotten
- Maggot-infested
- Excrement
- Putrid
- Rancid
- Noxious
- Vomit

- Infected
- Hairy
- Festering
- Repulsive
- Nauseating
- Stomach-churning
- Toxic
- Vile

Sorry – but I did warn you it was going to get uncomfortable!

Write down your new improved, disgusting Revolting Thing in as much
detail as possible here. Remember to use ALL your senses – how does it
look, feel, smell, sound?

_____

_____

_____

_____

_____

Focus on that thing, very closely. Close your eyes and think about it, feel it through your body and form a picture in your mind of you with this Revolting Thing that you wouldn't eat even for a million dollars. Imagine seeing it, picking it up and bringing it up to your mouth. Taste it, noticing how it makes you feel, especially in your stomach.

Write down below what you saw in your mind:

1) Is the picture you see in your mind black and white or colour?

_____

2) Is it close to you or far away?

_____

3) Is it bright or dim?

_____

4) Is it moving like a movie, or flat like a framed painting?

_____

5) Do you see yourself in the picture, or are you looking at the scene through your own eyes?

_____

OK, so now's where the rubber hits the road. This is where we associate your subconscious reaction to the Revolting Thing to your chosen Nemesis.

When I asked you to make a picture in your mind and answer the five questions, there will be some differences between your Nemesis and the Revolting Thing. All you have to do now is make the picture in your mind match the Revolting Thing when you think of your Nemesis. It's really easy and I'll share with you my Coke example to show you how.

Oh, I should probably check you haven't just eaten?

No?

OK, good - read on!

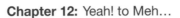

	<u>Nemesis</u>	<u>Revolting Thing</u>
	Coke	**Dog faeces dissolved in sump oil**
Question 1)	Colour	Black & White
Question 2)	Far away	Close
Question 3)	Bright	Dim
Question 4)	Moving (fast)	Moving (slow)
Question 5)	Own eyes	Own eyes

The next step is really very simple. What we do is:

1) Create a picture in our mind of us with the Nemesis BUT

2) Use the characteristics of the picture from the Revolting Thing.

For me, I thought about Coke, but in my mind I saw the picture as:

- Black and white.

- Far away from me.

- Dimly lit.

- Moving slowly.

- Through my own eyes (same for both).

This is the quick, simple way to imprint my subconscious reaction to the revolting thing onto my reaction to Coke. When you do this with an NLP Coach, it will be slightly more involved, but the principle is exactly the same. Check out **outsmartsugarnow.com** if you're interested in taking this further with some personalised coaching just for you.

Now that you know what my Revolting Thing was, can you see why it's now so easy for me to say "No, thank you!" to Coke??!! Do you want to go back and revise your Revolting Thing, now that you know what mine was?

To make it even easier for you to do this exercise on your own, here's some space to write down your answers side by side:

	Nemesis	**Revolting Thing**
	_____	_____
Question 1)	_____	_____
Question 2)	_____	_____
Question 3)	_____	_____
Question 4)	_____	_____
Question 5)	_____	_____

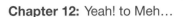

Now, think about your Nemesis, but make the picture in your mind match your answers to the Revolting Thing. It might take a couple of goes for this to stick, but once it does, you'll never feel the same way about your Nemesis again!

The Colour Con Shortcut

Well, you knew there was going to be a shortcut, didn't you? I think you know me well enough by now to know what to expect!

Simply by changing the colour of foods can impact how much you eat. We know certain foods are supposed to be green, like spinach, Granny Smith apples or broccoli. However green signifies that it might contain poison or mould in other foods – like white potatoes or cheddar cheese. Blue very rarely occurs naturally in food – the only one I could come up with is blueberries, which are really more purple than sky blue. Your brain doesn't recognise blue food as safe or healthy to eat, so use this to your advantage.

As Richard Dean, an NLP expert, says: "Turn that Mars Bar green or blue in your mind and you're likely to eat half as much". Probably a bit less confronting than my "Yeah to Meh…" process, but sometimes you need to start out gently!

CHAPTER 13

QUANTUM QUESTIONS

"Successful people ask better questions, and as a result, they get better answers."

— Tony Robbins

CHAPTER 13

QUANTUM QUESTIONS

"Affirmations are about as helpful as making a wish when you blow out your birthday cake candles."
— Tara Mitchell

A lot of people think affirmations are the most important tool in creating a positive mindset. I don't mind them, as they do help point your attention in a specific direction, but they're mildly effective at best and can actually be de-motivating at worst. I know this might sound a little counter-intuitive at first, but hear me out. If your subconscious doesn't believe what you're "affirming" consciously, the little so-and-so can sabotage you so its view of the world is maintained. Remember, it's all about safety for your unconscious mind – and often "safety" means staying exactly where you are, even if it's detrimental to you. Just ponder on these few affirmations I found on a weight loss site as an example, with the likely subconscious responses:

Conscious Affirmation: I nourish my body with healthy foods and enjoy exercising daily.

Subconscious: "Pfffffffft!! What about that ice-cream you had last night and the chocolate bar you thought no-one saw you eat at morning tea? I saw you though. And exercise? You HATE exercise with a passion!! Stop saying these silly things!"

Conscious Affirmation: I am beautifully sexy and slender.

Subconscious: "You don't look like a Victoria's Secret Model, so how can you call yourself sexy and slender? You'll never look like one either – what a dumb thing to say!"

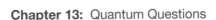

Conscious Affirmation: My body reflects what an extraordinary and unique person I am.

Subconscious: "Oh dear - got tickets on ourself, have we? There's nothing extraordinary or unique about you - everyone in your high-school class has gone on to do amazing things, but what have you achieved? Yeah, your body reflects that alright!"

Your subconscious can be a nasty piece of work sometimes – I know mine has! You may have noticed that affirmations look to an ideal future, but the sentence is stated in present tense. The idea is your mind believes the positive outcome is already happening now, and instructs your body to act accordingly. Sounds perfect in theory, right?

In practice, affirmations are really quite one-dimensional and, quite frankly, no more effective than making a wish on a star or blowing out birthday candles! You're simply stating what you want, which is great, but there's no instruction for your mind to follow up on or action. Who is the only person in the world that's going to make this happen for you?

That's right - You!

Let's break down that first affirmation above:

"I nourish my body with healthy foods and enjoy exercising daily."

Who's going to provide and eat the healthy food?

You.

Who's going to perform the exercise?

You.

Who's going to make sure you do it daily?

You.

We humans have managed to outsource most things, but despite what the late-night infomercials would have you believe, I'm pretty sure exercise is one we still have to do ourselves! But nothing in the affirmation actually helps you take ACTION towards those fantastic goals of eating healthily and exercising daily.

So what will you say instead of an affirmation to propel you towards massive ACTION? Well, I'm glad you asked!

Asking the right question is the single most effective way to get what you want and propel your life forward. Taking a moment to stop, determine your ideal outcome, and craft a great question which gets you that outcome is incredibly powerful and, quite simply, magical. So let's start with how we construct excellent questions.

The "Five W's" are, fortunately, not clones of George W Bush! They form part of the framework for learning languages and they ask open-ended questions, or ones that can't be answered with just "yes" or "no". These will help us in designing awesome questions and drive us forward to action. They are:

• Who…?

• What…?

• When…?

• Where…?

• Why…?

Add an "H" in there and you have the recipe for creating a punchy news story that all journalists use.

• How...?

I've devised a way to take this concept of asking questions and adding rocket fuel to make them 'Quantum Questions'. These are the questions that will create a Quantum Leap in your thinking and actions. Quantum Questions are like affirmations on steroids – they work on many levels to Outsmart your negative inner voice. There are certain ways to ask your Quantum Question and, despite there being five "W's" available to you, I find it's always best to avoid "Why" questions? Why? Because a WHY-NY question will always result in a WHINY-ME!! Let me explain...

Asking "Why" may seem on the surface to be helpful, as in a practical sense it means you can uncover all the things that need addressing and come up with a plan to overcome them. Sounds sensible right? And very scientific too, given that scientists' main mission in life is to find out "Why" things are the way they are. I don't know about you, but I'm not a qualified scientist (although I must say one of my best days at high school was when our chemistry teacher let us lose on the Oval with some lumps of pure sodium and a bucket of water. Explosions and much squealing of teenage girls ensued. The boys totally stayed super-cool, but you could tell they were just itching to squeal with joy too. But I digress...) and I'm not interested in an in depth psychoanalysis of why you're scoffing an entire family block of Dairy Milk in one sitting. I want you to move forward. Quickly and Easily.

Asking "Why" questions won't move you forward and, if you start asking ones like the examples below, you'll feel very disempowered very quickly:

- "Why can't I resist doughnuts and always eat the whole box before it gets back to the office?"

- "Why can I never stop at just one square of chocolate?"

- "Why does the whole tub of ice-cream disappear before I know it?"

- "Why can't I say "no" to that extra helping of cake, even though I know I'll feel bad afterwards?"

Why are these so disempowering? Because you bet your nasty little subconscious mind is gonna come up with a whole bunch of reasons Why! Like:

- "Because you're weak…"

- "Because you're pathetic…"

- "Because you have no self-control…"

- "Because you're not smart enough to know better…"

And then your deeper subconscious will start contributing, and that's where the real trouble starts:

- "Because you use sweets as a substitute for the love you didn't receive as a child…"

- "Because no-one cares if you get fat…"

- "Because you're overcompensating for the lack of control you feel at your job…"

- Because you failed Maths in school and have been failing in life ever since…."

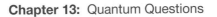

Oh dear.

If you ask a question of yourself, your brain is primed to keep going until it finds the answer and as much supporting evidence as it can uncover. Just like a trashy tabloid magazine reporter, it will keep digging until it uncovers all your buried, subconscious reasons for behaving the way that you do. We want to avoid that spiralling down into the depths of the "Poor Me" quagmire and ramp up your thought process.

OK – but what about a positive "Why" question? I still think these are short-sighted at best. For example, "Why am I healthy?!" is not the worst question in the world. It presupposes that you are already healthy (which puts your brain into a positive state) and your mind will go looking for things that prove you are indeed, healthy. This is a good thing.

But we want better than good! We want something that will propel you forward and get your subconscious working overtime to ensure you really do think that you're healthy and take all the actions necessary to keep you that way well into the future. So, what could we could do with this question to make it future-proof?

Here's how – ask a Quantum Question!

Let's start with a few examples:

"How can I eat even more healthily today?"

This will send your subconscious scurrying to unearth reasons why you're already eating healthily (answer + supporting evidence), but also look into the future to find other things you can actually do today to eat even more healthily. This will propel you forward and focus your mind on finding more answers and taking more action. Asking this question every day will keep the habit going.

"Who else can I spend time with today who will help me eat more healthily?"

I think this one is particularly important – Jim Rohn, business philosopher and entrepreneur, says "You are the average of the five people you spend the most time with". Stack the odds in your favour and surround yourself with people who are already where you want to be! This doesn't only refer to real life situations – if you're online, why not seek out people, websites and resources that can help you Outsmart sugar? Try **outsmartsugarnow.com** for a start!

"What other foods that I love and taste great that have no sugar can I eat today?"

You will set your brain a mission to find those foods and prime yourself to look forward to eating them. As you know from reading the "Dirty Marketing Tricks" chapter, your brain can easily imagine all the sensory experiences that come from consuming a food when prompted – so let's prompt it to look in all the right places!

"Where else can I find help to create amazing meals and snacks?"

You get the picture!

My personal favourite Quantum Question is

"What else can I do today to Outsmart Sugar?"

Even though it still appears to be a fairly simple question, the addition of "else" after "what" really shifts your current conscious thinking, as well as sending your subconscious off like a heat-seeking missile! You are effectively telling yourself that you're already doing SOMETHING (even if you haven't actually defined it) which shifts your brain into a positive frame After all, everyone likes to know we're already on the

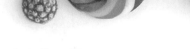

right track, don't we? It also sets your mind on a mission to find even more good stuff you can do. Isn't that fantastic?!

I really think this is one of the most powerful questions you can ask yourself in any part of your life…

"What else can I do today to…

> **…have more fun?**

> **…make more money?**

> **…expand my circle of friends?**

> **…be more loving to my partner/kids?**

> **…find more inner peace?**

> **…change the world?"**

I really encourage you to take this and run with it. Practise your Quantum Question daily and read them out loud. I know you might feel a little bit silly doing this at first, but there's some real science behind this (and you already know I love science, especially when it involves explosive action!). Let me give you a demonstration.

Think about how people get your attention. Do they pass you a note with your name on it? Well yes, they might sometimes – but we're past high school now aren't we? Would they be more likely to call out your name? Would you pay immediate attention to someone who called out your name? Of course you would. Indulge me and try a little exercise, just so I know you really get this. I think you'll find this fun!

Call out your own name, but only in your mind.

How much attention did you give it? Just a little? Did it even manage to cut through all the other inner talk and chatter that was going through your mind at the same time? I'm guessing probably not.

Now, call out your own name – out loud. Really LOUD!

Did you sit up like a meerkat on patrol? Did you look around to see who called you? Seems silly to do so, doesn't it? You know it's you doing the shouting! I still look around every time, even though I've been demonstrating this trick for years! Did you notice all of the inner talk and chatter just stopped, even if it was only for a second or two?

Interesting, isn't it?

You can now see the power of speaking out loud to yourself. I know talking to yourself is seen by some as a sign of madness, but isn't there a creative genius in madness? I find this technique profoundly genius – it can take years and years of meditative practise to silence the inner talk. Now you know all you have to do is shout your own name out loud to get an instant result! I think you now understand how important it is to read your Quantum Question out loud. Your conscious and subconscious minds are trained from a young age to respond to the spoken word and it's most powerful when it comes in the form of your own voice.

Now – let's get creative! Write down some of your Quantum Questions here and then choose a favourite to write out on a card and stick it up on your bathroom mirror, in your car or wherever you'll see it daily. I'll give you some help with the first three:

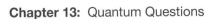

What else can I do today to _____?

Where else can I find more people to connect with about_____?

Who else can I spend time with to make me feel more _____?

Your turn!

_____?

_____?

_____?

_____?

_____?

_____?

_____?

There's one more type of Question I'd like to introduce you to. Yes, you guessed it - another short-cut!

If you find yourself ill-prepared for a situation – perhaps you've stumbled in on a party before preparing your "When I… Then I… responses that we formulated together in 'Personal Policy Making 101'. Here's a very quick Short-Circuit Question that will automatically have your brain look for the "right" decision.

"What would Batman do?"

Think of someone you respect and admire when it comes to healthy eating – perhaps it's an athlete, an actor or even someone in your own life that you look up to. Perhaps it's Sarah – that friend you have who never misses an opportunity to take the stairs and always takes her coffee black, no sugar thanks.

When you're faced with the easy option of a chocolate bar versus the healthy option of seeking out fresh fruit, rather than mindlessly grabbing the chocolate bar, stop and ask yourself:

"What would Sarah do?"

I'm pretty sure she'd head down the street to find an apple or banana – not only getting closer to her 10,000 step challenge for the day, but making the best choice to fuel her body.

Write down the names of at least three people and why they're an inspiration to you:

1)_____

...inspires me because...

_____

_____

_____

2)_____

...inspires me because...

_____

_____

_____

3)_____

...inspires me because...

_____

_____

_____

Now, choose the most inspiring and write their name below to create your very own Personalised Short-Circuit Question:

"What would_____do?"

CHAPTER 14

THREE PRINCIPLES TO LIVE BY

"You better cut the pizza in four pieces, because I'm not hungry enough to eat six."

— Yogi Berra

CHAPTER 14

THREE PRINCIPLES TO LIVE BY

"An ounce of preparation is worth a pound of snacks!"
— Tara Mitchell

I do love Yogi Berra's quote for this chapter – not only is it clever and amusing, but also a classic example of how we like to trick ourselves when it comes to food. We've already learned a whole lot about how to reprogram our brain, so now I want to share with you how to easily alter your physical environment to Outsmart Sugar.

There's pretty much just Three Principles to live by. When you take these on and utilise them in your everyday life, I guarantee you'll see massive changes to your sugar intake.

Principle 1) Out of Sight, Out of Mind

It's a well-known proverb and a bit of a cliché, but believe me - it really works! Once something is out of your line of sight, you'll forget about it and it's impossible to mindlessly reach for it. Remember we talked earlier about not even thinking about sugar? This is a neat little way to trick your brain into thinking there's no sugary foods available to you.

But if you do have sugary foods visible – watch out! My favourite Professor, Brian Wansink, says he can predict your weight just by looking at what you have on your kitchen counter, displayed on open shelves or sitting on your desk. After studying the contents of people's homes and offices (with their permission of course!) and recording their weight, this is what he found:

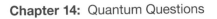

- Got sweet biscuits out on your kitchen bench-top? You're likely to weigh almost 4 kilos more than someone who doesn't.

- Do you have boxes of highly-processed, sugary breakfast cereal stacked out in the open? Your weight is almost certainly 8.5 kilos more than someone who has a more nutritious, non-processed, high protein breakfast.

- Here's the killer for me – soft drink lined up in a highly visible area means you're likely to be a whopping 11.3 kilos heavier than someone who doesn't. Don't you feel like dumping all that sugar water down the drain right now?? I can personally vouch for this one – jettisoning the brown sugar water from my life saw me drop two dress sizes, with absolutely no effort on my behalf at all! Soft drink is completely devoid of nutrition and the sooner you can turn your back on it, the better.

So clear all that crap out of your line of sight – now! "But what am I going to do with all that spare bench space?" I hear you ask. The good Professor has some exciting news for you on that front. His research also found that having fruit displayed prominently means you'll probably weight about 2 kilos LESS than someone who doesn't. Sounds to me like a great reason to dust off that big ol' fruit bowl you got for your 21st birthday, give it pride of place on your kitchen bench and fill it with beautiful, fresh seasonal fruit, don't you think?

What else could you do either at home or work to apply the Out of Sight, Out of Mind Principle? Write down your ideas here:

_____

_____

_____

Principle 2) Degrees of Difficulty

Here's a fun little piece of trivia for you: there are three calories in a single, plain M&M. Doesn't sound like much, does it? If you were to eat just one every now and then, it probably wouldn't have much of an effect. But no-one eats just one at a time! How any do you think you'd eat if someone laid out huge bowls of them, all over your office? Just ask Google! They used to scatter bowls of M&M's all over their offices – just one of the many, many things they do to keep employees happy and creative, such as pinball machines in the kitchen and slippery-dips replacing some staircases (really!).

In an experiment, Google placed lids on all the bowls of M&M's in their New York office. Lifting off a lid to get to chocolate doesn't seem like much of an effort, yet the results were dramatic. Three million (yes, MILLION!) less M&M's were consumed in that office in just one month!

Comprehending three million of anything is tough, so I'll break it down in a way that shows exactly what the cumulative effect of mindless eating can do to you:

• Google's New York office employs around 3,000 people.

• 3,000,000 M&M's divided by 3,000 employees = 1,000 M&M's per employee a month.

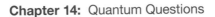

- 1,000 M&M's x 3 calories each = 3,000 calories.

- 3,500 additional calories per month = 1 pound (around 1/2 kilo) weight gain

Add that all up over 12 months, and just mindlessly grabbing tiny chocolates can lead to a weight gain of up to 6 kilos!

Introducing Degrees of Difficulty into accessing sugar is a really smart move. Simply putting a lid on an open bowl had a massive effect on Google consumption of M& M's. I'm sure you can find ways to incorporate escalating Degrees of Difficulty into your surroundings.

What could you do to introduce Degrees of Difficulty either at home or work? Write your ideas down here:

_____

_____

_____

_____

_____

_____

Principle 3) The Five P's

You've probably heard this popular military adage before (if you're feeling a little mischievous, you can add in the word in brackets to make it a Six-P Principle!):

Prior Planning Prevents (Piss) Poor Performance

"Be Prepared" is an excellent motto to live by – just ask any Boy Scout or Girl Guide! Planning and Preparation is the key to having control over every situation where you previously might have been tempted by sugar. Now, when I say "Be Prepared", I'm not asking you to spend hours every day getting ready for every single conceivable situation you might be faced with. That would be completely overwhelming and not a smart use of your time!

You can't control other people and you can't always control your environment, so simplifying your efforts into areas that you CAN control is the key to Outsmarting Sugar. I've discovered there's really only two areas to focus your preparation on:

1) **Automate Your Response to Offers of Sugar.**

2) **Have Alternative, Pre-portioned Foods Readily Available.**

Targeting just these two alone will eliminate having to think too hard and will reduce your Decision Fatigue significantly. Let's go into a bit more depth on both of these so I can show you just how easy it is to "Be Prepared".

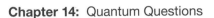

1) Automate Your Response to Offers of Sugar

We covered automating your responses in Chapter 8 by formulating your very own Personal Policies – turn back to have a look at what you wrote there to remind you. You might like to reflect on how far you've already come!

The "When I… Then I…" formula we worked on there is very powerful, but I have a confession to make. There's an even easier way to automate your response to offers of sugar that I haven't shared with you yet. Sorry about that. Actually… no I'm not – think of it as your reward for committing to reading this far in the book! Ready?

Here goes:

Just Say "No".

Actually, please say "No, thank you".

I like to think you're someone with manners and good graces! Saying "No, thank you" thoughtfully and with a certain level of charm is important when you're replying to others. No-one likes their offer to be rejected, so in the interests of preserving relationships, please use your manners! It's even more critical when talking to yourself. You'll remember from Chapter 11 on Inner Talk that being kind to yourself will positively impact on your emotional state.

Just using these three little words as your go-to response can have a huge impact on your sugar intake. Here are just a couple of situations where saying "No, thank you" will go a long way to Outsmarting Sugar:

Tea and Coffee

Many people claim they don't eat a lot of sugar, but mindlessly stir in a couple of teaspoons in every tea or coffee they drink. Think about this next time you're asked "one lump or two?" in your hot beverage:

- Every teaspoon of sugar contains 15 calories.

- Two hot beverages a day with one teaspoon of sugar each = 10,950 calories a year.

- Excess 10,950 calories a year = weight gain of 1.4 kilos.

Just by saying "No, thank you", you eliminate the possibility of sneakily gaining 1.4 kilos a year!

The Combo Deal

You already know how bad soft drink is and you've eliminated it from your kitchen at home. But sometimes you're caught in a food emergency and takeaway is the best you can do right now. That's OK – never feel bad about getting stuck with only one choice, just make sure you optimise that choice.

Have you noticed that pretty much every takeaway joint (both the multinationals and your local family-owned store) will offer some kind of deal that includes a soft drink? That's because they know everything tastes better with... Sugar (if you automatically used a certain brand name there, you now know exactly how effective their marketing is!). It can even improve the taste of second-rate, deep-fried, fish-of-questionable-origin from the crappiest fish and chip shop around!

The big problem with soft drink in combo deals is the huge amount of liquid calories it adds, mostly in the form of fructose. Unfortunately,

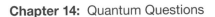

these calories don't flip the "I'm full" switch in your stomach and you won't save half your meal to eat later to compensate, will you? Let me put it to you this way: a small soft drink contains about the same amount of sugar you'd find in four apples. Would you be able to eat four apples AND a hamburger? I'm guessing not!

By just saying "No, thank you" to soft drink in your combo meal, you'll cut out a huge amount of sneaky sugar. Most places will be happy to substitute a bottle of water for the soft drink. Automatically selecting water as your beverage of choice also reduces your Decision Fatigue.

The Bread Basket

Eating out at a fantastic restaurant is one of life's great experiences for me and if there's a particularly spectacular dessert on the menu, I may well have it! Food should be celebrated and enjoyed, not stressed and guilted over, particularly at a fine dining establishment. So I'm not going to tell you to say "No, thank you" to dessert when you're eating out. However, if you habitually order dessert, even when you're just eating out for convenience, you may not even be aware of why you do it!

You're being primed right from the moment you sit down and that bread basket gets plopped down in front of you. But why is this a problem? Bread doesn't contain that much sugar, does it? Not always, but white bread behaves almost exactly the same way as refined sugar once it's digested. So that gives you a sugar rush, perfectly setting up your sugar-crash for the end of the meal, just in time for… dessert!

So just say "No, thank you" to the bread basket at restaurants. Oh, and when you get to the end of your meal, waiters know that if just one person at your table says "Yes please!" to dessert, the rest of the table will almost certainly order too. Watch next time you're dining out and I'll bet you see this phenomenon in action. If I really don't want dessert, but feel like I should order something to be sociable, I'll go with peppermint tea.

It's great for digestion and you still get the "closing ceremony" around finishing your meal.

2) Have Alternative, Pre-portioned Foods Readily Available

Investing just the smallest amount of effort here can have a massive pay-off. Food Manufacturers want you to believe you have no time to eat healthily and you should buy their sugar-laden, pre-packaged foods so you can spend more time with your family. Yeah, right – more quality family time is totally their motivation! (Sorry, my sarcasm has snuck in again!) What I find really quite sad is that, despite all these huge increases in "time-saving" convenience foods, most families don't sit down and eat together any more. Everyone's completely glued to their electronic device of choice, and this is one of the biggest reasons why we overeat.

Your stomach is actually pretty useless at letting you know when you've had enough, because it takes around 20 minutes to register feeling full. Your brain relies on visual clues to tell you when you're done eating – this is usually signified by an empty plate (or empty ice-cream tub!). When you have a distraction, like watching TV or surfing the web, your brain has no idea whether you've had four handfuls of M&M's or five, nor does it have a clue how full the bag was when you started. This is why you'll end up eating over 15% more if you're preoccupied whilst eating.

You shouldn't have to pay Food Manufacturers for convenience, especially when it's so easy to create it yourself! There are plenty of great ideas on **outsmartsugarnow.com**, but for now, here are a couple of my favourite quick tips to having great choices on hand:

- Even when you're eating well, accidentally overloading on healthy snacks can derail your good intentions. Pre-pack nuts, seeds and dried fruit into zip-lock bags or small containers to manage portions. These can also become part of your "Smart Snack" tubs below.

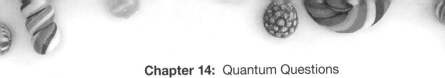

- Design your own "Smart Snack" tub and fill it with tasty, healthy snacks that you love, so you'll always have something on hand when you're hunting for a snack. Below are some of the things I like to have on hand at all times. You might like the sound of these, or you might come up with some even better ones, just for you!

Fridge Smart Snacks Tub

Hard-boiled eggs

Greek yoghurt

Berries

Dips – check the label for sugars, or make your own

Cut vegetables

Whole or pre-cut fruit

Tomato or vegetable juice

Cheese

Olives

Home-made snack bars. **Outsmartsugarnow.com** has some great ideas!

Pantry/Desk/Car Smart Snacks Tub

Nuts

Seeds

Dried Fruit (small amounts only – it's high in natural sugar!)

Nut butters. Again, check the label for sugars or make your own

Dark chocolate – at least 80%

Flax or seed crackers

Protein bars – be very cautious & check ingredients carefully

Canned tuna, salmon or sardines

Popcorn

Seaweed snacks

What will you keep in your Smart Snack tubs?

_____

_____

_____

_____

_____

_____

_____

_____

- Create "Smoothie Packs" to keep in the freezer. Smoothies are still my favourite breakfast of all – they're fast, portable and an easy way to get a couple of serves of fruit and vegetables into you early in the day. Hang on – did you say vegetables? Yep, that's right – no more ice-cream for me! Get on the Green Smoothie bandwagon and you'll already be ahead of the game before you even leave the house. Rather than deciding what you want in your smoothie each morning and

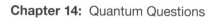

fussing about with a whole lot of different ingredients, pre-package them up ready to go and – Hey Presto! – you've reduced your Decision Fatigue again.

My Simple Starter formula for the perfect Green Smoothie is below. I've listed a few suggestions for each ingredient type to ease you in gently – you can get more adventurous later on if you want. I highly recommend increasing veggies and decreasing fruit as soon as you're accustomed to the taste. Using mild-tasting greens like baby spinach means you'll barely taste the "green" - I promise!

For One:

- 1 packed cup leafy greens (baby spinach, kale, beet leaves)

- 1.5 cups fruit (banana, mango, berries, pineapple)

- 1.5 cups liquid (water, coconut water, green tea)

- 1 scoop protein powder

- 1 tablespoon booster of your choice (chia seeds, nut butter, flax seeds)

Seal the first two ingredients in zip-lock bags and freeze. Make up a week's worth of these packs, so you're ready to go every morning. Then just pop them in your blender with the other ingredients, blend 'til smooth and you're good to go. Faster than ordering a muffin and coffee and more portable than sugary cereal and milk in a bowl!

I've found that starting your day with a great breakfast means you'll continue on that path all day. Your brain is already primed to target the best food choices for you and it will seek them out automatically for you. This helps reduce Decision Fatigue again, because unhealthy choices don't even make it onto your radar. That makes the rest of your day so much easier – and who doesn't want that?!

Remember my Three Principles to Live By:

Principle 1)   Out of Sight, Out of Mind

Principle 2)   Degrees of Difficulty

Principle 3)   The Five (or Six!) P's: Prior Planning Prevents (Piss) Poor Performance

Personalising your physical environment for each Principle will massively reduce your Decision Fatigue, as well as support all the clever methods and tricks you've learned throughout this book.

FINAL WORD

"The best time to plant a tree was 20 years ago. The second best time is now."

— Chinese proverb

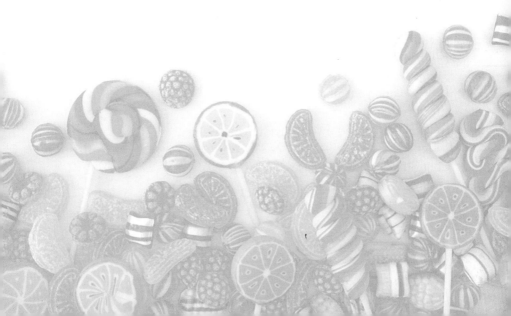

FINAL WORD

"Why 'Quit' sugar when you can simply Outsmart it?!"
— Tara Mitchell

So you've made it to the end of the book – congratulations and thank you! We've spent a lot of time together now and you know a whole lot more about me than you did when you first picked up this book. I truly hope you know a lot more about yourself now too!

I've shared with you a bunch of techniques, methods and tricks I've learned and developed, which have helped me tremendously – not only with Outsmarting Sugar, but also with other areas of my life. So what was your favourite? Was it:

- Getting your Lizard Brain on a leash?

- Understanding why Willpower doesn't work and what does?

- How to get a burst of self-confidence in three seconds?

- Knowing how to defend yourself against advertisers?

- How to tame your Inner Child?

- Breaking down and reconstructing your Habits?

- Controlling your emotions?

- Reducing Decision Fatigue?

Final Word

- Going from Yeah! to Meh…?

- Formulating Quantum Questions?

- Learning the 3 Principles to Live By?

Maybe it was something else entirely? Perhaps you'd like to write down your greatest learning or "AHA!" moment here:

_____

_____

_____

Whatever it is, you'll find that it now manifests in your life easily and effortlessly. You have all the resources you need at your fingertips and you'll find even more at **outsmartsugarnow.com**!

You've learned that our bodies were never designed to handle the amount of sugar that's now all too easily available, but you also know why we're programmed to seek it out. You now have some amazing tools to engage the awesome power of your mind and it is my hope that you use these to add incredible value to your life.

My wish for you is that, whatever you end up taking from this book, you live life to the full and make the most of every opportunity. Enjoy the best food, the best company and the best fun there is to have! Please remember that food is not something to be obsessed over, but created, shared and enjoyed with love and celebration. After all, truly experiencing the spirit of human bonding over authentic, wholesome food is one of life's greatest pleasures!

Living your life means reflecting on the past but not living in it – you can't change history, but you CAN change how you think, feel and visualise it! Life is measured by the actions you take and in the end, all that ultimately matters is what you've done. Not what you've said, or promised, or intended. Your defining moment is right now and your path will be decided by the very next step you take.

What's your next move?

Whatever move you choose, make it a Smart one!

Hugs and best wishes to you!!

Tara xxx

AUTHOR PROFILE

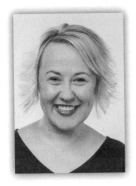

Tara Mitchell

Author, Entrepreneur, Life Coach, and Neuro-Linguistic Programming Trainer

Tara is an author, journalist, entrepreneur, life coach, Master Ericsonian hypnotherapist, and highly sought-after Neuro-Linguistic Programming trainer.

Her entrepreneurial spark ignited at the age of 14, when she started her first business making and selling Happy Pants to her classmates. She also began her love affair with writing and public speaking whilst still in school, reporting for the school newsletter and captaining the champion high-school debating team.

Prior to focusing her talents on assisting others with improving their lives, Tara qualified as an economist, graduating from The University of Adelaide and going on to earn a Graduate Diploma in Administration. After deciding against boring people to death for a living, Tara became a Wine and Spirits Educator – gaining a Graduate Diploma in Wine Business Management and an International Advanced Certificate in Wine and Spirits. This has afforded her all kinds of fascinating experiences, from teaching whiskey appreciation to the staff at London's finest hotels, hosting a Riesling and Cornish Pasty breakfast atop a high-altitude vineyard in the Clare Valley, and driving a sponsored pace car in the Tour Down Under cycling race.

Tara has an adventurous spirit that has motivated her to work and travel around the world. She managed a ski chalet in the French Alps, served lunch to royalty at Lord's Cricket Ground, danced on a float at the Notting Hill Carnival and bungee-jumped, para-sailed, scuba-dived and hot-air ballooned her way around the globe. As a published journalist, she managed to combine her love of music and writing to gain access to exclusive interviews with many world famous pioneers of electronic dance music across Europe and Australia.

Practicing what she teaches, Tara kicked a multiple-can-a-day Coca-Cola habit and weaned herself off ice-cream for breakfast (yes, really!). She is also a self-described recovered shopaholic, even making an appearance on the Today Tonight show where she demonstrated how changing her thinking got her out from under a mountain of credit card debt.

When she finds herself at home, she spends time atoning for her Happy Pants sins by creating much more beautiful clothing, as well as pretending to be a chef, engaging in light home renovation, reading and exercising her green thumb.

Tara now focuses on using her many talents to help others be more successful in all areas of life.

Tara Mitchell is the author of "Outsmart Sugar" and lives in Melbourne, Australia with her partner Toby.